The New Mom's Survival Guide

ALSO BY DR. JENNIFER WIDER
Published by Bantam Books

The Doctor's Complete College Girls' Health Guide: From Sex to Drugs to the Freshman Fifteen

The New Mom's Survival Guide

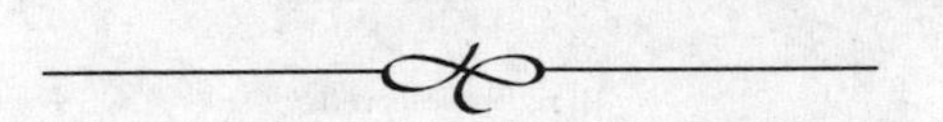

How to Reclaim Your Body, Your Health, Your Sanity, and Your Sex Life After Having a Baby

JENNIFER WIDER, MD

BANTAM BOOKS

THE NEW MOM'S SURVIVAL GUIDE
A Bantam Book / July 2008

Published by Bantam Dell
A Division of Random House, Inc.
New York, New York

Book design by Helene Berinsky

The information in this book is of a general nature and is for reference purposes only. It is not intended as a substitute for the medical advice of a physician. Readers should consult a physician in matters relating to health and particularly with respect to any symptoms that may require diagnosis or medical attention.

Library of Congress Cataloging-in-Publication Data
Wider, Jennifer.
The new mom's survival guide : how to reclaim your body, your health, your sanity, and your sex life after having a baby / Jennifer Wider.
p. cm.
ISBN 978-0-553-80503-1 (trade pbk.)
1. Mothers—Health and hygiene—Popular works. 2. Postnatal care—Popular works. I. Title.
RG801.W72 2008
618.6—dc22 2007043434

Printed in the United States of America
Published simultaneously in Canada

www.bantamdell.com

BVG 10 9 8 7 6 5 4 3 2 1

For my dad

Who has brought more than 5,000 lives into the world.
Your professionalism, integrity, and compassion
embody the very essence of being a doctor.

and

For my mom

My personal survival guide.
Your selflessness, encouragement, and unconditional love
embody the very essence of being a mother.

ACKNOWLEDGMENTS

Writing a book while raising young children can be a bit of a challenge, so I have more than a few people to thank. First off, thank you to my husband and my rock, Erez, who has continuously supported me through several manuscripts, late-night and early-morning radio shows, and reading my articles in *Cosmo* magazine (publicly). Your patience, kindness, and encouragement mean so much.

A special thank-you goes to my daughter, Orly, who is by far my biggest fan and who recently told me that she'd buy all my books in the bookstore if they languished on the shelf for more than two days. Your creativity, artistic abilities, and love of learning continue to inspire me.

And another special thank-you to my son, Ryan, whose afternoon nap allowed me to finish this book. Your curiosity and cleverness are a joy to watch develop. Thanks, too, to *The Very Hungry Caterpillar*, *Curious George*, and *Really*

Rosie videos that gave me a few extra minutes when Ryan woke up.

Being a mommy to both of you makes me a better person.

Thank you to all of the new moms who shared their experiences with me. A sincere thank-you goes to Lisa, Emily, Macon, Jamey, Annie, and our fearless leader, Karen B.—the original Brooklyn mommy group. And thank you to Laurice, who was always there to go through so many first year challenges with me.

Thank you to Susan Arellano who recognized the need for this book. And, finally, I'd like to thank Beth Rashbaum, whose tireless efforts and extraordinary editing abilities helped to make this book a reality.

CONTENTS

INTRODUCTION

When I was pregnant with my first child, I had absolutely no idea what to expect. I went about my business as if nothing was different. At work I'd occasionally glance down at my growing belly as thoughts of chubby, quiet, smiling babies dressed all in white filled my mind. I had convinced myself that my life wouldn't really change.

Fast-forward to after delivery—I was sitting in my infant daughter's room and we were both crying. She was crying because she needed a new diaper; I was crying because I missed my old life, felt wiped out from lack of sleep, and was simmering with resentment toward my husband, whose life hadn't really changed at all. To add insult to injury, he came home that night "in the mood." Was he on drugs?

Two months later, just as my daughter turned three months, I started a support group for new mothers. We were thrilled to be new mothers (most of the time), but we were also filled with raw, mixed, and overpowering emotions. And although each discussion always began with our children, the conversation eventually veered back to us.

We spoke about our sex lives, or lack thereof; our emotional state; the changes in our bodies, which we feared were permanent; our issues about staying at home versus going back to work, and oh so much more. Each week there was a new topic, and when the women found out that I was a doctor, the conversations shifted to our physical health: "Is it normal that my hair is falling out?" "Why can't I lose the weight?" "Why are my feet larger; will they ever shrink to their normal size?" "If my child has the croup, can I get it?" "When will it stop hurting to have sex?" "Ever since I had my son, when I laugh, urine comes out—is that normal?" We had all spent the nine months of pregnancy strictly monitored by a staff of medical professionals; but once the baby came, we were dropped like hotcakes. Even our families stopped asking how we were feeling! It became apparent to me that women have health issues that extend well beyond the birth of a baby, and questions that need answers. Just because we'd each had a baby, it didn't mean that our minds and bodies had ceased to exist.

There was no single resource available to us that could credibly answer our questions. And the resources that do deal with this period tend to focus on the health of the baby, not the baby's mother. If Mom is mentioned anywhere outside the epilogue, it is usually only in the context of postpartum depression. But new moms have many other health concerns that are particularly likely to arise at this time.

I remember at one of our support group sessions, a woman had spotted a skin change under her arm, and after going online, she came in crying hysterically, convinced she was dying from skin cancer. She didn't realize that certain skin changes were normal during and after pregnancy. What she had spotted turned out to be a normal skin tag.

As a doctor and a mother, I knew I had to do something. So I set out to write a book that could offer new mothers sound and reassuring medical advice about their physical and mental health. I interviewed a multitude of new moms to find out what issues were relevant to their lives. What I found was that given the time and opportunity, new moms have a lot to say.

Women are the caretakers for their families. They are responsible for the health and well-being of their partners, their children, and often their aging parents as well. But sometimes their own health issues can get lost in the shuffle. My hope is that I have created a solid, well-researched health guide for new moms that addresses their concerns about themselves—those concerns that tend to get buried in the avalanche of information about the health of their children.

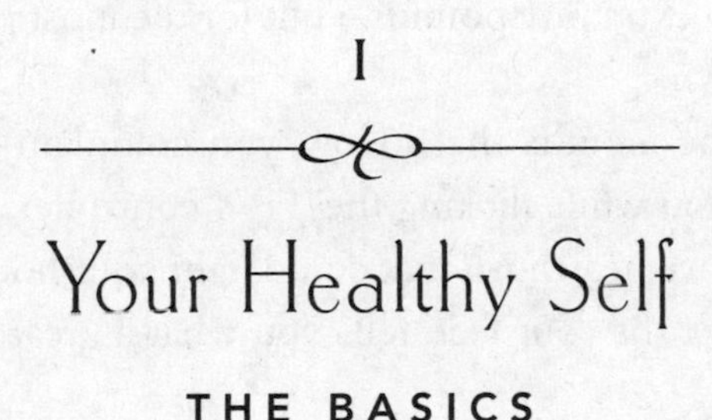

I

Your Healthy Self

THE BASICS

You've got to love your husband. He has sex, he has an orgasm, ejaculates, and nine months later calls himself Dad. You have sex, probably without an orgasm; for the next thirty minutes you lie propped up on a pillow with your legs in the air, hoping his sperm will make its way up the cervical canal and meet up with your egg; and then you wait anxiously until you can take a pregnancy test to find out whether in nine months you'll be able to call yourself Mom. Of course, all of this assumes you had planned to get pregnant, which doesn't take into account the percentage of pregnancies, however welcome they may be, that are unplanned.

But that's just the tip of the iceberg, right? You spend the next few months nauseated, vomiting, and eating saltines. All the while, he takes clients to four-star restaurants and eats four-course meals. While your body contorts into different shapes, his body stays exactly the same. Maybe he gains a few extra pity pounds—but for the most part, you're on your own.

Over the months that follow, you complain—a lot. He comforts you while flicking the TiVo controller. You burp, fart, and have heartburn that could light your house on fire. He smiles, rubs your feet, tells you what a great job you're doing.

When you get to bed, you can't sleep; he sleeps like a baby. Your mind is racing: *Will I be a good parent? What will our lives be like? How will I cope?* Maybe you even wake him out of his sound sleep with your questions. "Piece of cake," he tells you, and falls fast asleep again. You gaze down at your enormous belly, your aching breasts, the spider veins that are slowly creeping their way up your legs. You look at his body as he snores and realize that nothing's changed for him; is this fair? Do I even need to answer that question?

I always hated those husbands that told people, "We're pregnant." What do they mean, "we"? Are they kidding? *We* are NOT pregnant. If men could get pregnant *we'd* become extinct, and it wouldn't be gradual, either. It would be sudden, like an explosion, and nine months later, the human race would cease to exist.

All right, I'm running away with myself—but just a little.

It doesn't end there, though. After the baby comes out, your husband's body is still normal, but yours has gone through a war. You're breaking out and having mood swings like a teenager. He's trying to help but looks a little scared, and not of fatherhood, mind you—you think he might be scared of you! You look in the mirror; why wouldn't he be scared of you? Your feet are large, your hair is falling out, you haven't slept, and you're leaking from every opening in your body. Then, you gaze down at your sleeping baby and take a deep breath, while your husband hands you a cup of chamomile tea, and you know it's all worthwhile. That doesn't mean, however, that there aren't a lot of changes to be reckoned with, physical and emotional, and challenges to be overcome.

This book was written to help you learn how to take care of yourself after having a baby, and to let you know when you need to go to a doctor or other health professional when self-care isn't enough. With everybody's focus on the baby, it's easy for Mom to be forgotten. But if you're not well, physically or mentally, your baby will suffer too. Your baby needs a healthy mother. Taking care of yourself is a crucial step in learning how to take care of your family.

WHAT'S UP WITH MY SKIN?

I don't know about you, but I miss that "pregnancy glow." People used to come up to me left and right to tell me how good I looked and how much pregnancy agreed with me. After giving birth, however, it became abundantly clear that pregnancy had taken a toll on my skin. The glow was replaced by acne, stretch marks on my body, and spider veins on my legs. Friends complained of varicose veins and skin tags too. On top of the sleepless nights and stress which could make even a china doll break out, we were plagued by feelings that we'd never look as good as we had before we got pregnant. Here's the scoop on some of the top skin concerns and what you can do about them.

Acne

Why am I breaking out like a teenager? I'm a mom, for goodness sakes.

Unfortunately, being a mom won't protect you from your hormones, which have been on a roller-coaster ride lately. Acne during pregnancy is not uncommon and can linger after the baby's born. Surging hormone levels are responsible for an increase in oil-gland production, which can make the skin a breeding ground for zits. So if you thought your pimples ended with high school graduation, think again!

How come my girlfriend has the clearest complexion of all time and I look like a pimple-product commercial?

The same reason why she had heartburn during pregnancy and you didn't: We're all different. Some women will have acne and others won't. If you've suffered from acne in the past, especially during your period, it is more likely you will have acne during and after your pregnancy. There is some good news, however: Nursing may protect your skin from breaking out. Another good reason to breastfeed.

Will it ever go away?

Yes, acne will disappear for most women when their hormone levels normalize, usually within a few months. If you have a history of breaking out prior or during your menstrual cycle, you can expect the same pattern once you stop breastfeeding and your period resumes. But look on the bright side: At least you don't have to go to the senior prom with a pimple on your nose!

What can I do about those pesky zits in the meantime?

Remember back when Mom told you not to pop them? The same advice still applies. Do not touch or squeeze your acne—you can get a nasty infection which is the last thing you need right now.

Take care of your skin and keep it clean. Dermatologists recommend washing your face with a mild cleanser twice a day. Over-the-counter products which contain benzoyl peroxide and/or salicylic acid should be safe if you're nursing; just check the label. If the problem is really bad, you may need a prescription. Make an appointment with a dermatologist, and make sure the doctor knows you're nursing before he or she prescribes any medication.

Stretch Marks

Before getting pregnant, everyone warned me about stretch marks. What are they and why do we get them?

Stretch marks are one of those unwanted little gifts of pregnancy. Because that growing baby made your uterus expand so much, your tummy's skin paid the price. Stretch marks are reddish, slightly depressed streaks that are seen on the abdomen and occasionally on the buttocks, breasts, and thighs.

They appear because the elastic tissue in your skin gets

worn down as it stretches and grows with your pregnant body. Pregnant women aren't the only people blessed with stretch marks. Anyone experiencing rapid weight gain is at risk too, including bodybuilders, overweight and obese people, and even kids going through puberty.

Does everyone get them?

No. There are (very lucky) women out there without a single stretch mark on their bodies. Studies show that roughly fifty percent of women have stretch marks during and after their pregnancies.

Your stretch mark risk goes up if you are carrying more than one baby, have a large baby, or gain weight rapidly.

When will they go away?

Do you want the good news or the bad news first? Let's start with the bad news: They won't really go away. But, here's the good news: They'll fade. Stretch marks fade significantly by six to twelve months post-pregnancy. So instead of those lovely reddish streaks, you're left with a silvery white remnant. Just consider it a battle scar from pregnancy!

Can I prevent them from happening to me?

My mother-in-law says yes. She swears by cocoa butter and bought me a tub of cream to slather all over myself during my first pregnancy. After my clothes repeatedly got stuck to my stomach and thighs, I did some research. The real answer is no. (I didn't have the heart to tell her and re-gifted the second tub of cream during my second pregnancy to an unsuspecting relative!) No cream or lotion has been medically proven to help. So don't waste your money.

Varicose Veins

Help! I have large, twisted, blue veins running down the back of my calves.

Welcome to the club that no one wants a membership to. You have varicose veins, enlarged, cordlike veins that often take up residence in your legs. Let's be honest: They're not so pretty. They often conjure up images of Grandma in a bathing suit.

Why do we get them?

Pregnant women are vulnerable to varicose veins for several reasons. Pregnancy increases the amount of blood in your body and the blood can pool in your legs, making the veins larger. As your uterus gets bigger with the growing baby, the added pressure gets exerted on the veins in your legs. Plus, your hormones can relax the walls of the veins, further adding to the problem.

My legs ache; could it be the varicose veins?

Unfortunately, yes. To add insult to injury, varicose veins can cause pain, aches, a feeling of heaviness, and cramps. They can also cause itchiness and throbbing. These symptoms tend to get worse if you sit or stand in one place for an extended period of time.

Take note: If one leg becomes swollen, red, or painful, seek medical attention right away. You may have a blood clot and need to see a doctor immediately.

Is there relief for my symptoms?

Yes. Many doctors recommend compression stockings, which won't land you on the fashion pages of the newspaper, but will help ease your aches and pains. By compressing the flesh of your legs, they help get the blood moving more efficiently. Speak with your doctor and make sure the stockings fit properly. Getting the wrong size isn't going to help, especially if the stockings are too big.

I thought the varicose veins would disappear after I gave birth. But mine haven't. What's up with that?

Most varicose veins will improve within three months post-pregnancy. But some will linger. If yours are sticking around and causing unpleasant symptoms, it's time to see a doctor.

What's the treatment for varicose veins?

Good news: There are many different treatments for varicose veins. From surgery to injections to lasers, you have a host of different options. And you have many different types of doctors to choose from as well: Plastic surgeons, interventional radiologists, and dermatologists all perform these kinds of procedures. Discuss the options with your primary doctor to see which one is right for you. Remember, all procedures can have possible side effects, so discuss these as well.

Spider Veins

I noticed red, branching blood vessels on my legs—what are these?

They're called spider veins, another battle scar of pregnancy. But don't despair: They usually fade quite a bit post-pregnancy.

Why do I have them?

Spider veins are thin veins that lie close to the surface of the skin. They show up when you're pregnant because of the increase in blood circulation. They're also caused by hormonal changes. Some experts believe that crossing your legs while sitting can bring them on because the blood in your legs gets backed up. There's also good evidence that they are inherited, so if Mom has red spiders running up and down her legs, chances are: so will you.

Are they similar to varicose veins?

Sort of. Spider veins are smaller than varicose veins, but they both show up during and after pregnancy. Varicose veins can be painful and may worsen over time. Spider veins are generally not painful and fade or disappear post-pregnancy.

It's been over a year since I gave birth and my spider veins haven't disappeared; what can I do?

There are several treatments available. Many women opt for sclerotherapy, a procedure in which the vein is injected with a solution that makes it collapse, and as a result, it becomes less noticeable. Laser surgery is also available. Both treatments may have side effects including swelling, pain, and bruising. Make sure to discuss these and other related matters with your doctor.

Also keep in mind that while most veins don't disappear completely, the procedures usually cause them to fade considerably.

Melasma or "the Mask of Pregnancy"

What is melasma?

Melasma, often called "the mask of pregnancy," is discolored patches of skin on the face. It's caused by the overproduction of melanin, a pigment that gives your skin its color. It commonly affects the cheeks, nose, and forehead. The condition is linked to your body's hormonal changes and can show up during pregnancy or when you take oral contraceptives or undergo hormone replacement therapy.

Is it common?

Yes. Melasma is very common and affects roughly six million women. Women with darker skin tones are more likely to get it. Important to note: Sun exposure can heighten your risk for melasma—so limit your tanning time and make sure to use sunblock with an SPF of at least fifteen.

I've had my baby, why hasn't the melasma gone away?

For most women, melasma will fade several months after delivery. For others, it can persist. Some women report having melasma for many years post-pregnancy; others report that their melasma never went away at all. The not-so-good news: Even if your melasma does go away, it may come back in subsequent pregnancies.

Can I treat it?

Although there is no cure for melasma, it can be effectively treated. Creams containing hydroquinone have been shown to help fade the patches of melasma. Chemical peels and topical steroid creams have been shown to work, as well as laser treatment. Remember, many treatments have side effects, so you should definitely consult a dermatologist.

Skin Tags

Help! After I had my son, I noticed several small pieces of skin hanging down from under my breasts; is this normal?

Yes, it's normal. You have skin tags, which commonly develop after pregnancy or as people age. They're totally harmless and often show up in the folds of your skin. Your neck, breasts, and armpits are common hot spots.

Will they go away on their own?

Unfortunately, the answer is no. Your skin tags are here to stay. Skin tags do not resolve after pregnancy.

Can they turn into skin cancer?

No. Skin tags are not precancerous and will never turn into skin cancer. They shouldn't cause you any discomfort unless they're located in an area of friction, like under a bra strap, at which point, the tags can become red and inflamed, itchy, and even painful.

I hate the way they look; can I get rid of them?

You sure can. Some women opt to have skin tags removed for cosmetic reasons. Others eliminate the ones that get easily irritated. Dermatologists can cut, freeze, or burn them off, and the procedure is usually quick and virtually pain-free. Don't ever attempt to remove them yourself. You could cause an infection, blood clot, or bleeding.

Cherry Hemangiomas

I have these little red moles on my stomach and back. What are they?

It sounds like you have vascular growths known as cherry hemangiomas. They are smooth, small, red bumps that can grow slightly larger with time. They get their name from their color and are formed from the growth of dilated (enlarged) capillaries and small veins.

Are they dangerous?

No. You can relax. Cherry hemangiomas are totally benign and will never change into anything scary.

Why do I have them?

Cherry hemangiomas affect both men and women. They become more common as we age. There is some evidence that they are associated with hormones, making pregnancy an opportune time to develop them.

Is there any treatment for them?

Cherry hemangiomas won't cause any physical symptoms. They will bleed, however, if they get scratched or cut. They can be removed for cosmetic purposes by laser or minor surgery. Speak to your dermatologist if you choose to remove them.

WHAT'S UP WITH MY HAIR FALLING OUT?

Have you been combing truckloads of hair out of your head? Does your bathroom floor look like the floor at your hair salon? If you've answered yes to these questions, don't panic! You are *not* going bald, I repeat, *not* going bald. Many women will experience substantial hair loss within one to four months after delivery. It's a normal part of a cyclical process. When you were pregnant, your hormones increased the growing hair phase (anagen stage) relative to your resting hair phase (telogen stage). So the body retained hair that would otherwise have fallen out normally and gradually. After the baby is born and the hormone levels change, however, you start shedding the extra hair. This abrupt hair loss is known to the medical community as *telogen effluvium.*

When will it stop falling out?

Relax, there is an end in sight! For the vast majority of women, post-pregnancy hair loss is temporary. The cycle of normal hair growth will kick in around six to twelve months. But be gentle. Avoid vigorous hair brushing, curling irons, braiding, or anything else that will put undue stress on your delicate hair. You don't want to do anything to increase your hair loss during this time.

It's been almost six months and my hair is still falling out; can it be something else?

It could be, especially if you have other symptoms. Thyroid disease is a common cause of hair loss and can be triggered by pregnancy. (See thyroid, p. 36.) You should make an appointment with your doctor. Iron-deficiency anemia, hormonal imbalances, and certain medications can cause hair loss in women. So, make sure to mention this to your doctor.

I'm totally embarrassed, but ever since I was pregnant I've had dark hair on my face and

upper lip that won't go away. What's wrong with me?

Nothing. Those same hormones responsible for hair growth are to blame. Some women experience mild hirsutism, or excess hair growth, in unwanted places including the face, breasts, and stomach. Don't fret: It will likely disappear a few months after delivery. Waxing or shaving is fine. If you want to bleach or use other solutions containing chemicals, consult your doctor, especially if you're breastfeeding.

If the hair growth is severe and doesn't go away within a few months, you may want to see your doctor, especially if you have other symptoms, including a deepening of the voice, irregular periods, and excessive acne. Other factors may be at play, including polycystic ovary syndrome or hormone-secreting growths.

WHAT'S UP WITH MY NAILS?

You gave up manicures while you were pregnant because you heard that chemicals in the nail polish could harm the baby. When you asked your doctor about it, she wasn't sure; but you wanted to err on the safe side.

You cut your nails often, because your pregnancy hormones made them grow quickly. You fantasized about the manicure/pedicure you were going to get after the baby came. But now, your nails seem brittle; they're peeling and don't look too healthy. That manicure seems out of the question.

My nails are a mess but my neighbor's look better than ever. What gives?

Some women notice changes in their nails during and after pregnancy. I've spoken to women who say their nails were stronger throughout their pregnancies; other women I've spoken to complained that their nails were flimsy and broke easily while they were pregnant. Most women will see a difference one way or the other.

Will my nails go back to normal?

Yes, you can go ahead and book that appointment at Nails Are Us. As soon as your hormones normalize, your nails will go back to the way they were before your pregnancy. If you are breastfeeding, your nails may not change back to normal until you stop.

Is nail polish safe while I'm breastfeeding?

It depends on who you ask. Studies in laboratory rats have shown that certain chemicals used to prevent chipping of nail polish, namely di-n-butyl phthalate (DBP), can cause birth defects. More research is needed to determine whether these findings can be applied to human beings. Also, more studies are needed to define the risks during breastfeeding. The jury's still out on this one, so proceed with caution!

WHAT'S UP WITH MY BREASTS?

Does this scenario ring a bell? You're nursing at 3 A.M. Your breasts hurt, the baby has fallen asleep on your nipple but you don't want to move for fear you'll wake her. After all, it's the only time she really falls into a deep sleep—when she's connected to your body.

You glance down at your breasts—are they really yours? They don't look the same anymore. They're not as firm as they once were; in fact, they're totally sagging. And how about those nipples? They're so large and they stick out so far, they look like they're from Mars.

What happened to my breasts?

They've been through a lot . . . your poor breasts. During your pregnancy, they increased in size, became more sensitive, and developed dark veins. Your nipples and areolas (the circular areas surrounding the nipples) darkened and got larger. They leaked and probably still do. For many of you, your breasts equal mealtime for the baby. They've been sucked, pulled, bitten, and twisted. So be grateful to them for everything they've endured.

I don't like way they look. Will they ever go back to normal?

Most likely, your breasts will return to their normal shape after you stop breastfeeding. But beware: There may be some subtle changes.

Many women complain that their breasts have lost their firmness. Some notice that the size of their breasts is smaller. Others don't see a difference. No matter which group you fall into, your breasts have been under the influence of hormones—so you can expect a few changes.

I'm like a leaky faucet; is there any way to lessen my milk flow?

All I can say is: Get used to it! There really isn't anything you can do to stop your breasts from leaking. One of my friends used to leak at the mere mention of anything to do with babies, including Pampers commercials. If this is you, make sure to carry a supply of breast pads everywhere you go. And if things are just as bad at night, line the bed with something so you don't wake up in a puddle!

I've stopped breastfeeding, but I can still express a milky fluid from my nipples. Is that normal?

Probably. Some women are able to express for many months after they stop breastfeeding. But be aware: Spontaneous discharge (fluid that appears without squeezing) should be looked at by a doctor, especially if you haven't breastfed for a while and are experiencing irregular periods or no period at all. A variety of hormonal conditions could be responsible and you should get it checked out. Also, any bloody discharge should be looked at by a doctor. But don't flip out. The vast majority of cases of nipple discharge are benign and nothing to worry about.

WHAT'S UP WITH MY VAGINA?

Okay, stop blushing! Every woman in the world has one and during your delivery it was the star of the show. But now things down there don't seem so stellar, so it's no wonder you are concerned about your vagina.

Your pregnancy took a toll on your vagina. Some of us had vaginas which grew to the size of a grapefruit from swelling and pushing out that cute (not so) little baby. Others had varicose veins popping out near their vulva and/or vagina. Some of us had episiotomies or vaginal tears. Most of us had an increase in vaginal discharge during the pregnancy, and vaginal bleeding after the pregnancy. So, needless to say, that vagina of yours has been on overdrive during the last year or so.

Ow! My vagina hurts.

Join the club, sister! If you had an episiotomy (an incision to help the baby get out), or if you had tearing (lacerations in the vaginal tissue), your vagina will likely be sore. In the immediate future, you'll need to take good care of the area. Use ice packs and cold cloths for the swelling. Keep the area clean and squirt a bottle of warm water on your vagina while urinating—to lessen the sting. Over time, this soreness will go away. Because everyone is different, the time to heal can vary—but you should feel a lot better about six weeks after delivery. If you don't, make sure you visit your doctor to rule out an infection around the incision.

Why am I still bleeding?

Everyone bleeds from their vagina after they give birth. In the very beginning, the flow is quite heavy. I like to call it "the Bionic Woman's period" because, although it is not a real period, the flow, which is a combo of sloughed uterine lining and blood, often resembles your period. The medical term for it is *lochia.* Over the next few days, the flow usually lessens and the color of the blood changes to a pinkish-red and then becomes a brownish color. For most women, it turns to a clear, yellowish discharge within a month. Others bleed for longer. If you are bleeding heavily or continue to pass clots for more than a few weeks, contact your doctor.

P.S. Wear pads. I know, I know—you hate them. So did I, but using tampons can put you at risk for a nasty infection. Plus, I don't know about you, but the thought of putting something back up my vagina at that point gave me the chills!

Why is my vagina so dry now that I'm no longer bleeding?

After the baby is born and the bleeding stops (around three to five weeks post-delivery), your vagina is actually quite dry. This is especially true if you are breastfeeding. You can blame your body's low estrogen levels. This is a large part of the reason why sex can hurt during this time period. If you're in the mood, go get a crate of K-Y Jelly!

My vagina is itchy and painful, and I've recently noticed some discharge. Is that normal?

No. It sounds like you may have vaginitis, or inflammation of the vagina. It can be caused by a host of things including: lowered estrogen levels, bacteria, and yeast. The most common symptoms are itching; redness; foul-smelling discharge (bacterial); white, cottage-cheese–like discharge (yeast); and pain while urinating. Although it's normal for many women to have vaginal pain and pain on urination for a little while after their pregnancies, the discharge suggests that you should see your doctor. You'll need to get treated if it is caused by bacteria or yeast.

I'm embarrassed to have sex. Will the varicose veins near my vagina go away?

Yes. For most women, varicose veins in the vaginal region will improve after the baby is born. The varicose veins appeared in the first place because the growing uterus put a ton of pressure on your pelvic veins. Once the baby is born, the pressure disappears and your varicose veins should improve. For women with a family history of varicose veins or overweight women, the veins may linger. If they are causing you pain, speak with your doctor about your options.

WHAT'S UP WITH MY FEET?

Was it just me or did your foot grow a size too? Before my pregnancy I was a size 7, now I'm a size 8. I had to throw out several pairs of my favorite shoes while my husband made bad jokes about Fred Flintstone.

It came to a head when my daughter was three months

old; we were going to a party at the beach—my first real outing since I had the baby. I tried to squeeze my feet into these hot summer sandals. No luck. After reenacting a scene from *Cinderella,* not only did I feel like the ugly, large-footed stepsister, I was crying louder than my newborn. I consoled myself the only way I knew how. I went out and bought myself three pairs of Jimmy Choos . . . size 8.

Will my feet shrink down to their normal size?

During your pregnancy, the body holds on to extra water and as a result, your feet can swell, making it difficult to wear your favorite shoes. But you assume your feet will shrink down to normal size once the baby comes, right? Wrong. When you were pregnant, hormones were released to loosen your pelvic ligaments so the baby could have an easier time traveling through the birth canal to make her debut. These hormones didn't stop with your pelvis, however; they left their mark on your feet, too. As a result, your foot ligaments relaxed and your little feet became a little wider. So while the swelling caused by water will go away after you have the baby, the changes to your ligaments are permanent. My advice: Think of your bigger feet as an excuse to get your husband to babysit while you go shoe shopping.

Is there anything I can do to prevent foot growth during pregnancy?

Probably not, but some women swear by orthotics, which are shoe inserts that can give more support to the foot and ankle. You should speak to a podiatrist about this if you're interested. And don't assume the worst: Some women don't seem to experience any permanent change in shoe size.

WHAT'S UP WITH MY PERIOD?

Remember those days when you were pregnant and didn't have to think at all about getting your period—or worry about not getting it? Not having a period was one of the best things about having that (not so) little bump. But now that the baby is here, and your period isn't, you've started worrying that you could be pregnant. And now you're wishing for that monthly friend that used to be such a drag to reappear in your life. *Come back,* you call in your sleep. *Please don't let me be pregnant again just yet.*

When will my period come back?

It all depends. I've spoken to women who got their periods right away and others who didn't start menstruating for many, many months. Studies reveal that menstruation resumes at an average of six to eight weeks after delivery in women who are not breastfeeding. For women who breastfeed, the period returns more slowly. The vast majority of women who breastfeed will have their period by thirty-six weeks. Some breastfeeding women report getting their period as early as two months, others report not getting their periods for up to eighteen months after delivery.

If I don't have my period yet, can I get pregnant?

YES! Two things happen during your menstrual cycle: The first is ovulation, or the release of an egg, and the other is the bleeding, or menstruation. While the two usually go hand in hand, it is possible in some instances to have one without the other. Your ovary can release an egg without bleeding, so it is possible to get pregnant.

Can breastfeeding protect me from getting pregnant?

It can, but you need to be careful; in fact, you need to be absolutely vigilant. The lactation amenorrhea method (LAM) involves using breastfeeding as a form of contraception. As the baby sucks, the hormones that get released stop the release of other hormones, which are the ones that facilitate and support a pregnancy.

LAM can be very effective but requires a large commitment from the mother and will only work if directions are strictly followed. The mom needs to breastfeed on demand with little to no supplementation. Her menses cannot have resumed and the baby needs to be less than six months old. This method usually requires nursing around the clock, at least six times a day.

If you are serious about using LAM for contraception, you should check with a lactation consultant to make sure you are following the guidelines properly.

My period is different since I had my baby—why?

I've heard this from a lot of women but couldn't find any scientific evidence to explain it. Some women complain that their periods got longer and heavier after the baby. Others told me that their periods were lighter. Usually, the first few periods after the baby tend to be heavier than normal. Your regular pattern should resume within the first year.

Help! My period is irregular and it's been months since I stopped breastfeeding.

First off, relax! Irregular periods are very common and most of the time, not harmful to your health. Most women will experience an irregular cycle at one time or another; after all, our bodies aren't machines.

Try to keep track of any changes you may be experiencing, because there are a host of different reasons you may have an irregular period which include:

- **Illnesses or infections:** Being sick or having an infection can disrupt or change your period.
- **Rapid weight loss:** Be careful—you may have dropped those pounds too quickly or you may be dieting too much.
- **Poor nutrition:** Make sure you are eating a well-balanced diet. A plate full of bean sprouts for breakfast, lunch, and dinner isn't good for your menstrual cycle or your body!
- **Overexercising:** If you're on that treadmill 24–7 or living at your gym, you may want to tone it down a bit!
- **Stress:** Believe it or not, emotional stress can have an effect on your period.
- **Drugs or supplements:** Certain medications and herbal remedies can affect your cycle.

- **Hormones:** All sorts of hormonal conditions can disrupt your period, including: thyroid problems, polycystic ovarian syndrome, and adrenal or pituitary conditions.
- **Uterine problems:** Uterine fibroids (growths), cysts, or endometriosis (the presence of uterine tissue in abnormal locations) can change your bleeding patterns.
- **Perimenopause:** Irregular periods are one of the hallmarks of perimenopause. Women who are entering menopause can experience heavy periods, and longer or shorter cycles.
- **Pregnancy:** Oops! If you think you could be pregnant again, buy a test.

If you experience one or two irregular cycles, don't worry. If it starts to become a pattern, see your doctor, who can help figure out the cause and, if necessary, the proper treatment.

WHAT'S UP WITH MY BOWEL MOVEMENTS?

Now we're getting into the nitty-gritty of the postpartum period. Painful bowel movements are, by far, one of the most unwelcome side effects of childbirth. And I have to admit, no one ever warned me how bad this problem can get. I shudder at the thought of my first bowel movement after my daughter was born. I was sitting in the bathroom at my parents' house for two hours praying for a normal bowel movement and asking myself how I could possibly push anything out ever again. My muscles felt like they'd retired and moved to

Florida. I was shaking and sweating and when it finally came, I felt like I was passing shards of glass. I almost passed out.

This doesn't happen to everyone, mind you. Many of my friends were spared an experience this grueling. But if you've had an episiotomy, prolonged labor with lots of pushing, and/or suffered from hemorrhoids during the pregnancy, chances are you'll have some degree of constipation and pain.

Why do you get constipated after the baby is born?

There are a number of possible reasons for constipation after delivery. If you had a vaginal delivery, all of that pushing can take a toll on your body. In the first few days to weeks, your body is exhausted, especially the muscles that you used to push out the baby. And guess what? They're the same muscles that you use to have a bowel movement. Your perineum, the area between your vaginal opening and rectum, is probably pretty sore, which makes the process even harder, especially if the tissue is torn or stitched up, because if you feel pain during a bowel movement you're likely to inadvertently hold it in, which can contribute to constipation. Pregnancy can put you at risk for hemorrhoids (enlarged veins in the rectum) which can up your chances of constipation. The problem with hemorrhoids is that straining to pass stool can worsen them—so it can become a vicious cycle.

Also, some of the medications you may have used to fight the pain during and after delivery can cause constipation, as can the iron pills you might be taking to treat blood loss and/or anemia.

How long does constipation last?

It all depends. For many women, the problem will go away in the first few days to weeks. But don't ignore the symptoms because constipation can linger for a long time if you don't manage it.

How can you treat it?

There are many ways to help ease constipation. Start by drinking eight to ten glasses of water a day. If you're breastfeeding, that's all the more reason to drink a lot of water and stay well-hydrated. Get up and move. Sitting for prolonged periods of time can make the problem worse. Don't forget to increase the fiber and roughage in your diet with food such as fruits, vegetables, whole grains, bran muffins, and cereal. I lived on prunes for weeks. I drank prune juice and ate dried prunes with all of my meals. And while it doesn't sound all that appetizing—it really worked!

If necessary, you may want to try a stool softener and/or laxative. Some people even need to use enemas. If you fall into this category, you should speak to your doctor about which medications are safe to use, especially if you are breastfeeding. For severe cases of hemorrhoids, a minor surgical procedure may be necessary.

Also, if you're taking iron supplements, speak with your health care provider about ways to help alleviate your constipation. There are several types of iron pills that are easier on the digestive tract.

What if it doesn't get better?

Don't worry, the vast majority of cases resolve. I know how you feel, though; I often worried that I was doomed to painful bowel movements forever. But the earlier you address the problem, the sooner it is likely to disappear!

For those of you experiencing constipation for weeks on end, speak with your doctor, especially if you have extensive rectal bleeding. The doctor can isolate the cause and rule out something more serious.

2

Your Healthy Self

DISEASES AND CONDITIONS TRIGGERED BY PREGNANCY AND LABOR

While the vast majority of women return to their normal selves soon after the baby is born, pregnancy and delivery can trigger a host of conditions and diseases that can affect you for months or even years beyond the birth. The changes of pregnancy can result in both short-term and long-term health consequences, many of which are easily treatable if diagnosed early on.

However, the life of a new mother is so filled with demands from the newborn that she may not even notice that anything is wrong. Perhaps you assumed your pale skin and racing heart were just the inevitable result of being a new mom, but in fact they may be signs of an iron-deficiency anemia. Extreme exhaustion, hair loss, and anxiety may be the result of a thyroid abnormality, not just the normal stress of the changes in your life.

The purpose of this chapter is not to alarm you, as—let me say again—the vast majority of women come out of pregnancy fine, without any serious health issues. But for the women who are affected, recognizing the signs and symptoms of these diseases and conditions is vital to their proper management and treatment. The conditions mentioned in this chapter range from mild to severe and from extremely common to rare. The take-home message is to pay attention to your body. Don't ignore symptoms that may be interfering with your daily life. Trust your instinct if something feels wrong and seek medical attention right away. Just because you're a mom doesn't mean your health and well-being should take a backseat to everybody else's. Paying attention to the red flags that may be staring you in the face will help not just you but everyone else in your family.

ORAL HEALTH PROBLEMS

Was it just me or did your mouth bleed like crazy after you brushed your teeth while pregnant? Even after brushing and flossing regularly, was your mouth still swollen and sore? At the dentist's office, did that sign that read, "If you ignore your teeth, they'll go away" make you wonder what you were doing wrong?

Can pregnancy affect a person's oral health?

You bet it can! Dental issues often arise during pregnancy due to elevated hormone levels. These high levels of hormones can make the teeth more susceptible to plaque and bacteria. The gums get red and swollen and bleed more easily. This is sometimes referred to as "pregnancy gingivitis."

Do the problems go away after delivery?

Not necessarily. Even after delivery, if a woman is nursing, the hormone levels remain high. This causes the same swelling and bleeding that she experienced during the pregnancy. Women who have had issues with their gums during pregnancy are more likely to experience problems afterward, according to Sally Cram, DDS, spokesperson for the American Dental Association.

What are pregnancy tumors in the mouth?

Some pregnant women experience the overgrowth of gum tissue, which can appear as swollen, red bumps between the teeth. It often shows up during the second trimester and is related to excess plaque. The overgrown tissue tends to bleed easily during and after pregnancy and does *not* usually resolve once the baby is born. It often requires surgical removal after delivery.

Are certain women at higher risk for gum problems?

Yes. Women who have issues with their gums during puberty and/or their monthly periods are more likely to experience problems during and after pregnancy. In addition, women who smoke, have poorly controlled diabetes, or have suppressed immune systems are more likely to suffer from gum disease.

Is gum disease serious?

It can be. Recent studies have shown a relationship between preterm babies and mothers with untreated gum disease, according to Dr. Cram. So, it's important to get the appropriate treatment during pregnancy. And remember, even if your baby was born at full term, untreated gum disease has also been linked to a heightened risk of heart and respiratory diseases. So before, during, and after pregnancy, you have good reasons not to ignore your oral health.

How can gum disease be prevented during and after pregnancy?

The American Dental Association recommends brushing twice a day with a soft toothbrush and flossing once. Avoid hard bristles, which can exacerbate the bleeding. See your dentist for regular cleanings and checkups during and after the pregnancy. If you have problems with your gums and are planning to get pregnant or are in the early stages of pregnancy, it may be wise to speak with your dentist about steps you can take to keep the problems in check.

ANEMIA

You haven't felt quite right lately. You're really tired, but it's more than that. Sure, you've been up late at night feeding the baby and you haven't slept more than three hours in a row for who knows how long. But you just don't feel like yourself, even your tired self. When your mom visited last week, she told you how pale you looked and that you needed some sun. You've also had several dizzy spells and noticed that your heart is racing a lot.

Are you imagining it or is something really wrong?

You're probably not making it up; women can usually tell when something isn't quite right with their bodies. It sounds like you may have anemia, a condition that occurs when your blood doesn't contain enough hemoglobin. Hemoglobin is a protein in red blood cells that carries oxygen to different parts of your body. The most common type of anemia in women is caused by a lack of iron in the body, which interferes with the production of hemoglobin.

How do you know if you're anemic?

Most people with anemia feel very tired and lack energy. Other symptoms include: pale skin, racing heart, dizziness, difficulty concentrating, shortness of breath, pins and needles or a cold sensation in the hands or feet, and possibly headaches.

For some people with mild anemia, there are no symptoms. As the condition worsens, the symptoms will show up.

Are pregnant women at risk?

Yes. Women in general are at risk for iron-deficiency anemia because of their menstrual cycle. When the body loses blood, it loses iron. This is especially true for women with heavy periods. Becoming pregnant can put a woman at further risk, because the developing fetus needs iron and will take what it needs from the mother. If Mom had low iron to begin with, pregnancy will exacerbate the problem and set her up for problems in the postpartum period.

Does childbirth put a woman at additional risk?

It definitely can. During delivery, women can lose a considerable amount of blood, resulting in significant iron loss.

Too many women walk around in a post-pregnancy haze, suffering from anemia for months on end without even realizing they have a medical problem. It isn't easy being a new mom, with physical and emotional demands that you've never experienced before. Add anemia on top of these challenges and it can become difficult to function.

How is anemia diagnosed?

If you suspect that you're anemic, see your doctor. Diagnosing anemia is quick and easy and can be done with a simple blood test. Other tests may be done to confirm the underlying cause.

What's the treatment?

If it's determined that you have an iron-deficiency anemia, you can be treated with iron supplements. Your doctor can help figure out the best course of action depending on the results of your blood test. Sometimes, adding iron-rich foods to your diet—red meat, lentils, green-leafy vegetables, and liver—can help, but again, your doctor should advise you.

What does my diet have to do with anemia?

It's important to note that what you eat can put you at risk for an iron-deficiency anemia. Women who cut meat out of their diets completely are particularly at risk. This is why it is so important to eat a well-balanced diet, especially while breastfeeding, a time when additional demands are being placed on your body. If you are a vegetarian or have other dietary restrictions, make sure to discuss them with your doctor or a nutritionist, who can help you create a nutritional plan that will help prevent you from becoming anemic.

THYROID

Do you feel tired lately? Who doesn't? And who even has the time to notice? It's pretty easy to forget all about yourself when you're so busy taking care of everyone else.

But suddenly you start to add up the things that don't seem quite right. Besides feeling like a truck ran over you, when you look in the mirror, you notice that your hair's falling out and you have huge black circles under your eyes. In the past, you've always been able to shed those extra pounds, but now the diet you've been on isn't working. You feel down, every little thing is making you cry lately, and you don't know why. You ask your friends and they tell you: It's all normal. After all, fatigue, depression, weight problems, and hair loss are supposedly "normal" for a new mother.

Is it normal?

Maybe. But maybe not. You may have a thyroid problem called postpartum thyroiditis, which literally means inflammation of the thyroid gland after giving birth.

What is the thyroid gland?

The thyroid gland is part of the endocrine system and is located underneath your larynx, or voice box. It is the largest gland in the neck and is shaped like a butterfly. The gland produces thyroid hormones, which help regulate metabolism, growth, and many other processes in your body. These hormones play a key role in the cellular activities of the body.

What happens to the gland after giving birth?

In some women, the thyroid gland gets inflamed and goes a little haywire after the birth of the baby, producing either too much hormone (hyperthyroidism) or too little hormone (hypothyroidism). The enlarged, inflamed gland is known as a "goiter," and can often be felt by touching the neck. Why this happens in certain women and not in others is yet to be determined.

Are thyroid problems common in women my age?

Thyroid problems are quite common in women after they give birth. In fact, as many as ten percent of all new mothers may suffer from postpartum thyroid problems. It's often missed because thyroid conditions can be easily confused with "tired mother syndrome," which afflicts virtually all new mothers.

What are the symptoms?

Typically, a woman with postpartum thyroiditis will experience symptoms of hyperthyroidism first and then hypothyroidism a few months later. Some women find that their symptoms fluctuate back and forth.

The symptoms of **hyperthyroidism** can include:

- nervousness or anxiety
- racing heart
- feeling excessively warm
- inability to concentrate
- weight loss
- difficulty sleeping

The symptoms of **hypothyroidism** can include:

- weakness or fatigue
- depression
- headache
- constipation
- memory loss
- dry skin
- hair loss
- weight gain or the inability to lose weight
- intolerance to cold temperatures

As you can see, these symptoms are pretty vague and often seem typical of what women experience in the weeks and months following the birth of a child, especially the symptoms of hypothyroidism. I mean, what new mom isn't exhausted or having problems shedding those extra pounds?

Will it go away?

For the majority of women, postpartum thyroiditis is a temporary condition which will go away by itself within a few months. However, roughly twenty-five to thirty percent of women who develop postpartum thyroiditis will develop permanent hypothyroidism within five years after they deliver.

What is the treatment?

Here's the good news: Most women don't need to be treated. Many women feel relieved just knowing the cause of their symptoms and the fact that their discomfort will likely go away within a few months. Others will need to be treated with hormone replacement therapy.

How would I know if I needed to be treated?

You wouldn't—that is, not without being told by a doctor. So, you should definitely seek medical attention if your symptoms persist. Your doctor should do a complete medical history and physical exam. Tests may include a simple blood test to check your thyroid hormone levels or possibly a radioactive iodine uptake test, if hyperthyroid symptoms are present.

If I have thyroid problems in one pregnancy, am I at risk in subsequent pregnancies?

Yes. Women who experience thyroid problems with one pregnancy are more likely to experience them in future pregnancies. It's important to note that women with insulin-dependent diabetes are also at a higher risk for postpartum thyroiditis. Make sure to alert your doctor to your medical history, especially if you've switched physicians. Your hormone levels should be monitored with blood tests after you give birth.

Can thyroid problems interfere with breastfeeding?

Most women with thyroid disease can breastfeed, but you should definitely consult your doctor. In women suspected of hyperthyroidism, radioactive iodine scans may be necessary, and if a thyroid problem is confirmed, the treatment may also involve radioactive iodine. Any exposure to a radioactive substance means you will have to wean the baby, at least temporarily. Certain medications are okay while you are breastfeeding, but others may not be, so a medical professional will best be able to guide you.

LOSS OF URINE

It's been six months since you had your son, and your "little problem" isn't going away. You went to a dinner dance with your husband last night and sneezed during one of the slow dances. You couldn't believe it when you noticed that you had wet your pants. You ran to the bathroom to check and sure enough there was a spot of urine on the back of your dress. You were mortified and left immediately. You've been doing the exercises that your doctor recommended, but it doesn't seem to be working.

Why is this happening?

You are experiencing urinary incontinence, the accidental loss of urine from your bladder. This problem affects millions of women in the United States and despite the fact that pregnancy and birth is one of its most common causes, it isn't often discussed as a possible side effect of pregnancy.

There are many commercials about stress incontinence—is this the same thing?

There are several different types of urinary incontinence, and stress incontinence is the most common. It is characterized by the loss of urine when a person exerts pressure or stress on her bladder by coughing, sneezing, lifting something heavy, or even laughing. It affects women much more often than men.

Isn't this something that just happens to elderly women?

Although it's most common in women over the age of fifty, several recent studies have shown that more women experience urinary incontinence after their pregnancies than previously thought. The problem usually occurs right after pregnancy, but one study revealed that more than a third of the women polled were still losing urine one year after they gave birth.

How does pregnancy cause it?

The extra weight of pregnancy can weaken your pelvic floor muscles, which are located under your bladder. These muscles help keep the urethra, or the tube that carries urine from the bladder to outside the body, closed. When the muscles weaken, urine can leak out. Nerves also play a role in bladder control and can get damaged during delivery; the result can be the loss of urine. Some studies suggest that fluctuating hormone levels can also have an effect. Low levels of estrogen can cause the bladder-control muscles to weaken as well.

Will the problem go away on its own?

For most postpartum women, the problem will resolve itself. However, if you are still experiencing the loss of urine six weeks after delivery, you'll need to speak with your doctor, who will likely refer you to a urologist, or a physician who specializes in the urinary tract. It's important to note that incontinence can start up several months after you give birth as well. Whenever it occurs, don't ignore it.

How is it diagnosed?

There are many ways to diagnose urinary incontinence. The doctor will likely perform a physical exam which often includes a pelvic and rectal exam. You may be asked to keep a "voiding diary" to record how many times you urinate and when the leakage occurs. This can help the clinician zero in on the underlying cause.

Other possible diagnostic tests include:

- Post-Void Residual Measurement (PVR), a test that measures the amount of urine after voiding.
- Urodynamic testing, which involves a temporary catheter and X-rays to assess the storage function of the bladder after it is filled with fluid.
- Ultrasound, to image the urinary tract and pelvis.
- Cystoscopy, a scope that can image the inside of the bladder.

How is urinary incontinence treated?

There are many different treatments for urinary incontinence including exercises, vaginal devices, medication, and surgery. Treatment depends on the cause, and what works for one person may not work best for the next person. Your doctor will ultimately find what works best for you. Most women are successfully treated without surgery.

The doctor told me that it would go away on its own without treatment. Any tips for coping in the meantime?

Worrying about your own urine leaking is not exactly something you planned for as a new mom, so here are some ways to help lessen the problem until it resolves on its own.

- Rule out a urinary tract infection (UTI). If you have burning, pain, or urgency when you urinate, you may have a UTI. UTIs are sometimes the cause of incontinence and if this is the case, treatment with an antibiotic will clear up both problems.
- Use pads. It sounds simple enough, and the ones you use for your period will do the trick.
- Do Kegels. These pelvic muscle–strengthening exercises can definitely help. See the following section on pelvic prolapse for instructions.
- Cut out the caffeine. Lowering your intake of coffee and other caffeinated beverages may help. Some studies claim that caffeine can worsen incontinence in some women.
- No smoking. You can add cigarettes to the list of factors that may exacerbate urinary incontinence, giving you yet another reason not to smoke.

I'm too embarrassed to seek help.

You shouldn't be. This problem is very common and your doctor has undoubtedly treated it many times before. Urinary incontinence is very curable, so seek help for it immediately.

PELVIC PROLAPSE

After your third pregnancy, you've been experiencing pressure in your vaginal area. When you pick up the baby—who isn't that heavy, mind you—urine tends to leak out. In fact, it's been leaking out whenever you cough or laugh. You have the sensation that something is about to fall out of your vagina. Yesterday, you looked in a mirror, and saw a bulge of pinkish tissue coming out of your vaginal opening.

Did the doctor forget to take something out during the delivery?

Don't worry—baby, placenta, and the works are all out. But it does sound like you're experiencing uterine prolapse, a condition caused by weakening of the pelvic muscles and ligaments. When the muscles and ligaments holding up the uterus experience a significant amount of stress and strain, the uterus can actually sag and move down into the vaginal canal.

How does childbirth cause it?

Any stress placed on the pelvic muscles, including prolonged constipation, chronic coughing, and obesity, can cause uterine prolapse, but childbirth tops the list. The intense strain placed on the body during childbirth can damage the tissues and result in considerable muscle weakness. Uterine prolapse occurs most commonly in women who have had multiple vaginal births, prolonged and difficult labors, and/or deliveries that involved forceps.

How do you know if you have uterine prolapse?

You might not know it. Mild cases of prolapse don't usually produce any symptoms. But if your case is moderate to severe, you probably would realize something is wrong. The symptoms are unmistakable and can include: a feeling of pressure or pain in the vagina, lower back pain, urine leakage, frequent urination, chronic urinary tract infections, pain during menses and/or sexual intercourse, and a bulging of tissue from the vaginal canal.

P.S. Your uterus isn't the only organ that can prolapse in the pelvis. Bladder prolapse is another possibility and will usually cause the same symptoms.

What should you do if you think you have it?

Go see your doctor. If you're experiencing the symptoms that we've mentioned, it is more than likely your ob-gyn will be able to make the diagnosis with a pelvic exam. If additional tests are necessary to make the diagnosis, they might include X-rays and a voiding cystourethrogram, which uses dye and an X-ray video to monitor the ability of your bladder to empty its contents.

How is pelvic prolapse treated?

The good news is that this condition can be effectively treated. Do you remember what Kegel exercises were? Your doctor probably told you about them when you were pregnant. Guess what? These exercises can help strengthen your pelvic floor muscles and lessen the symptoms in many mild cases of prolapse.

For moderate to severe cases, a device known as a pessary can be used. It's rubber, shaped like a ring, and gets inserted into the vagina. It is used to prevent the uterus or bladder from sagging. Surgery is another option and should be discussed with your physician.

Remind me, how do you do Kegels?

Squeeze your pelvic muscles like you are trying to stop yourself from urinating, hold and count to five. Many doctors recommend doing this at least two hundred times a day. Don't get overwhelmed; you can do these in the car, while writing e-mails, or while watching your favorite movie. And no one will know what you're doing—it can be your little secret. Plus, as a bonus, they may enhance sexual sensation!

FECAL INCONTINENCE

You don't even want to admit it to yourself, let alone discuss it with anyone, but you're having a hard time controlling your bowel movements. You've been passing a lot of gas since your son was born and really didn't give it much thought. But last week, you accidentally soiled your pants and began to realize something was really wrong.

What's going on?

Some women suffer from fecal incontinence after they give birth. Most often, it involves passing gas uncontrollably. Less often, it involves the leaking of stool. This problem can be very embarrassing and many women have a hard time discussing it. Sometimes childbirth-related fecal incontinence doesn't manifest until years later, which makes the cause harder to figure out.

Why does it happen?

Fecal incontinence can occur after the delivery of a child for several reasons. It can result from a muscle injury to the ringlike muscles known as the anal internal and/or external sphincters. These muscles help keep stool inside, but if damaged, they can't perform properly and stool can leak. If the doctor used forceps during the delivery or performed an extensive episiotomy, or if there was a serious laceration or tear, the risk of muscle damage increases.

Fecal incontinence can also result if the nerves in that region get damaged during delivery. It can also result from pelvic floor dysfunction, a condition in which the muscles in the pelvic region that support the rectal area don't work properly.

How is fecal incontinence diagnosed?

Your doctor will likely do a complete physical exam and ask a variety of questions about your pregnancy, delivery, and past medical history. Medical tests may aid in the diagnosis and can include:

- Anal manometry: assesses the anal sphincter's ability to fully close and the function of the rectum.
- Sonogram: to image the structures of the anal and rectal areas.

- Anal electromyography: can test for nerve damage that may have resulted during childbirth.
- Proctography: can measure how well the rectum holds stool and how well it can void.

I'm on weight-loss pills. Could this be a side effect?

It's certainly something to consider. First off, you should definitely consult your physician if you are taking any medications in the post-pregnancy period, especially if you are breastfeeding. Having said that, certain weight-loss pills have been known to cause fatty stools or even fecal incontinence (another good thing to mention to your physician or health care professional).

Is there any hope for me or will it last forever?

Thankfully, for some women, the incontinence is temporary and will improve in time. In others, the problem refuses to go away and can actually get worse. Extensive episiotomies and severe lacerations that involve the anal sphincter muscles are more likely to cause long-term problems. If the problem persists, you should of course seek treatment.

What is the treatment?

The treatment is based on the underlying cause of the problem and how severe it is. Options range from diet modification to bowel training, medication, and surgery.

Surgery may be required for incontinence resulting from

a muscle injury. There are a variety of different surgical procedures available for this problem. Every case is different, so talking to your doctor will help you determine the best course of action.

What type of dietary changes can help?

You'd be surprised how much changes in your diet may help the problem. For some people, even small changes can make a world of difference.

- Make a record. Keep track of the foods you eat and write down when you have an episode of fecal incontinence. Common offenders include: dairy products, fatty or greasy foods, artificial sweeteners, spicy foods, alcohol, and caffeine. The goal is to determine which foods make your stool looser and cause diarrhea, so keep a thorough record.
- Space your beverages. Drinking fluid can speed the movement of food through the digestive tract. To put the brakes on this rapid passage, don't eat and drink at the same time.
- Don't eat large meals. Sometimes eating smaller meals more often throughout the day can help.
- Bulk up your stool. If you experience watery diarrhea, eat foods that add some bulk to your bowel movements. These include: bananas, rice, yogurt, peanut butter, and bread.

RHEUMATOID ARTHRITIS

Both your right and left wrists are stiff and have been aching lately and you can't figure out what's causing it. The pain seems worse in the morning and gets better as the day progresses. You were hoping it would just disappear, but it comes back day after day. Your fingers seem to be getting a bit stiff too. When you lift the baby, you feel a little weak, but maybe that's from lack of sleep?

What's going on?

Your symptoms sound a lot like rheumatoid arthritis, a chronic condition that affects women much more often than men. The disease often begins in women during their childbearing years. It can afflict any joint, but frequently starts in the fingers, hands, or wrists. It usually affects joints on both sides of the body, but occasionally affects the organs, including the skin, eyes, lungs, heart, blood, kidneys, and nervous system.

What causes it?

Unfortunately, the exact cause of rheumatoid arthritis is not known. Many believe that it results from an interplay of environmental, genetic, and hormonal factors.

Scientists *have* discovered that the immune system is involved and that's why rheumatoid arthritis is considered to be an autoimmune disease. In autoimmune conditions, the body's immune system launches an attack on the body. In rheumatoid arthritis, the lining of the joints get attacked, resulting in inflammation, swelling, and damage to the cartilage and joint. In some cases, various organs in the body can be the target of an immune attack.

Are there other symptoms?

In addition to joint pain and stiffness, rheumatoid arthritis can affect people in many different ways, causing fatigue, weakness, flu-like symptoms, nodules or lumps under the skin (usually in the hands), muscle pain, loss of appetite, swollen glands, and skin redness or inflammation.

Do women get rheumatoid arthritis more often than men?

Rheumatoid arthritis affects women two to three times more often than men, according to statistics from the National Arthritis Foundation. No one knows the reason for sure, but research is being done to help us arrive at a better understanding. Women seem to develop this type of arthritis in disproportionate numbers in the year following a pregnancy. Generally speaking, in women who have the disease prior to pregnancy, symptoms tend to get better during the pregnancy and worsen after delivery. More research studies are needed to fully understand the relationship between gender and rheumatoid arthritis.

How is it diagnosed?

You'll most likely be referred to a rheumatologist, or doctor specializing in conditions affecting the bones, muscles, and joints. There is no one test that can diagnose rheumatoid arthritis. The diagnosis is based on several things including a thorough medical history and physical exam, X-rays, and blood tests.

If you have any suspicion that you might have rheumatoid arthritis, keep track of your symptoms before you see the doctor because you may be asked to fill out a fairly extensive questionnaire at the office.

It is crucial to get diagnosed as early as possible, because early treatment may prevent some of the more serious complications of the disease, so don't dclay seeing a health care professional if your symptoms are like those described above.

What's the treatment?

There are a host of medications available. The treatment really depends on the individual. Since rheumatoid arthritis can affect people differently, the treatments need to be customized accordingly. If you're breastfeeding, make sure to mention it to the doctor before taking any prescribed drugs.

One last thing . . .

Try to stay positive. I realize that you have so much to deal with as a new mom and the last thing you wanted to add to your growing "to-do" list is a chronic condition. Just remember, early and proper treatment of rheumatoid arthritis has been shown to prevent permanent disabilities. Stay on top of your condition and you can be healthy and productive.

LUPUS

After you took the baby to the beach, you noticed a weird-looking rash on your face. It was red, blotchy, and covered your cheeks and the bridge of your nose, sort of like a mask. You thought it was a sunburn, but it didn't go away when you expected it to. Then, you spiked a fever of 101 degrees, which lasted more than a week, and you felt totally exhausted. You ignored it all until you woke up one morning with severe pain in both of your wrists. At that point, you knew something wasn't right.

What's wrong with you?

You may have lupus, a disease in which the body's immune system doesn't function properly and attacks healthy tissue. This can result in damage to various parts of the body, including skin, joints, kidneys, lungs, heart, and blood vessels. Some people have very mild cases while others have more severe cases. Most everyone with lupus is likely to have times when symptoms flare up, and other times when few to no symptoms are manifesting.

Lupus and other autoimmune diseases are much more common in women than men. Among women, African-Americans are more likely to develop lupus, as are women of Hispanic, Native American, and Asian descent.

Why did it show up now?

Cases of lupus seem to peak during the childbearing years and often show up for the first time during pregnancy or shortly thereafter. The precise cause of the disease is unknown, but many doctors believe that a mixture of factors including genetic, hormonal, and environmental play a role. Research studies have suggested that pregnancy hormones can influence the immune system and perhaps play a role in the course of autoimmune diseases, including lupus.

What are the symptoms?

The symptoms of lupus can vary greatly from person to person. They may come and go and will usually not appear all at once. The most common symptoms include: a malar (butterfly-shaped) rash across the cheeks and bridge of the nose, arthritis (which includes joint pain, stiffness, and swelling), unexplained fever, fatigue, nausea, vomiting, Raynaud's phenomenon (a condition where the body's extremities turn numb and pale when exposed to cold temperatures), and hair loss. In more severe cases, dizziness, vision problems, kidney problems, heart and lung problems, and blood vessel disorders can result.

Can the baby get it?

No. The vast majority of babies born to mothers with lupus are fine. A small percentage (roughly three percent) will get "neonatal lupus," but it isn't the same as the mom's lupus. Neonatal lupus usually manifests itself with a rash and abnormal blood counts. It will likely disappear in the first few months of the baby's life. Some infants born to moms with lupus have heart conditions, so it's important to follow up with the pediatrician.

How is lupus diagnosed?

The American Academy of Rheumatology has established criteria for diagnosing lupus. A person needs to have symptoms or lab results filling four of the eleven criteria in order to be diagnosed. To make the diagnosis, your doctor will take a full medical history and perform a complete physical exam. Lab tests can be used to look for antibodies in the blood and screen for abnormal blood counts.

How is lupus treated?

Because each individual case is different, treatment varies depending on the course of the disease. The medications used include: nonsteroidal anti-inflammatory drugs to reduce joint inflammation and swelling, steroids, and immunosuppressants to suppress the exaggerated immune response many people get with lupus. New treatments are currently being researched.

Does lupus interfere with breastfeeding?

It depends. Breastfeeding is possible for many women with lupus, but for some women, it isn't recommended. Certain medications, such as steroids, can lessen the milk supply. Other medications can cross into the breast milk and harm the baby. Consult your physician to discuss your individual case.

Having a baby is hard enough; how can anyone deal with being a new mom and having lupus?

It's true, adding lupus to the mix can be really tough. But plenty of women do it and you can too! The key factor is setting aside enough time to take care of yourself properly. Here are some tips that will make dealing with this additional challenge a little easier:

- See your doctor regularly. There's no excuse for skipping appointments. Take the baby with you, if need be, or find a babysitter or relative.
- Take all of your medications as prescribed. Be responsible and don't skip doses. Set up a schedule, if necessary. For example, take your medication before you feed the baby every morning.
- Get rest. You're probably laughing to yourself and thinking, "What new mom gets enough sleep?" But it's very important for women with lupus to get an adequate amount of sleep because studies show that lupus can cause severe fatigue. Maybe you can enlist your husband or a willing relative to take the night shift?
- Avoid the sun. Studies show that excessive sunlight can trigger a flare-up of lupus. Stay covered and protect yourself.
- Avoid smoking and alcohol at all costs. Bad for everyone, cigarettes and alcohol are worse for women with lupus because they up your chances of heart and kidney problems in the future.
- Exercise regularly. Exercising can help keep the flare-ups under control and help speed recovery time.
- Try to stay positive. Women with chronic diseases are at risk for depression. So if you're feeling down in the

dumps, it may be more than the baby blues—get the help you need!

CELIAC DISEASE

After you had the baby, you started having gas, and it's not the kind of gas you had during the pregnancy—this gas could fill up the Goodyear blimp. And it's so embarrassing. You were sitting in a mommy support group and the cramps were so bad, you couldn't hold it in. You sprinted to the bathroom and had diarrhea, the sixth bout that week! You've also noticed that your stool doesn't look normal, it's sort of pale. And that's not all. You've been exhausted and had some joint pain. You thought it was just typical tiredness, but your in-laws gave you a weekend away during which you slept eleven hours in a row for two nights, and you were still tired.

Is this just gas left over from pregnancy?

Probably not. Most pregnant women suffer from gas at some time or another. In fact, most people do. But as uncomfortable as it is, the problem usually resolves after childbirth, once the muscles in the digestive tract resume normal function. The gas described above, accompanied by bloating, chronic diarrhea, pale-colored stool, fatigue, and joint pain post-pregnancy, could point to something else.

What could it be?

If your symptoms present themselves consistently, you may have something called *celiac disease*, a digestive disorder that disrupts the absorption of nutrients from your food. People with this disease cannot digest gluten, a protein typically found in wheat, rye, and barley. If they eat food that contains gluten, the immune system launches a response that can damage the digestive tract and prevent absorption of nutrients like proteins, carbohydrates, fats, vitamins, and minerals.

Are gas and diarrhea the only symptoms?

No. There's a long list of symptoms. But remember, everyone is different; some people have most of the symptoms, while others have no symptoms or very few. Having said that, the symptoms include recurring abdominal pain, cramps, bloating, pale and funky-smelling stool, bone or joint pain, change in weight (up or down), fatigue, sores in the mouth, and an itchy skin rash.

Does pregnancy cause this disease?

Not really, but it can trigger it. Celiac disease tends to run in families. Besides pregnancy, other factors that may activate it include childbirth, stress, surgery, or infection.

Are certain people at higher risk?

While anyone can develop celiac disease, there are some risk factors worth mentioning.

- Genetics: Your risk goes up if one or more members of your immediate family has the disease.

- Ethnicity: Persons of European descent are diagnosed with celiac disease more often than other ethnic groups.
- Personal medical history of autoimmune disease: Women with diabetes, rheumatoid arthritis, lupus, or thyroid disease tend to be at greater risk for celiac disease.

How is celiac disease diagnosed?

Celiac disease is often underdiagnosed because the symptoms can be mistaken for a host of different problems ranging from indigestion to the stomach flu. Many people don't realize that something more serious is going on and neglect to see a physician.

If you have some of the symptoms described above, see your doctor, who will likely start with a blood test. If the results point to celiac disease, a biopsy of the small intestine can be taken to confirm.

What's the treatment?

The treatment involves cutting gluten out of the diet. Most doctors will recommend consulting a nutritionist who can help set up a gluten-free diet plan. For the vast majority of patients, this diet will ease the symptoms and let the digestive tract heal. Nowadays, there are a large range of products in the grocery store with labels that read "gluten-free." The diet can be challenging, but if you follow it, you should be able to avoid or alleviate many of the symptoms and lead a normal and productive life.

Any tips on how to cope with celiac disease?

As with other chronic diseases, being a mom and coping with celiac disease can be a challenge. But there *are* things you can do to lessen the emotional and physical burden that comes along with this type of diagnosis.

- Learn all about gluten. Educate yourself as much as possible about foods that contain gluten. It isn't always obvious and it has been known to show up in food additives, sauce thickeners, and vegetable proteins. Many times, restaurants will not know if certain meals have been prepared with gluten. In the United States, it is not required for food labels to indicate whether gluten is present or not. This can be frustrating, but you'll get the hang of it and the more you know, the better off you'll be.
- Get emotional support. Women who suffer from chronic diseases can experience more stress and emotional burden than other women. That's why it is vital to have a strong support network. Talk to your doctor about locating other people with celiac disease. Sometimes sharing stories, ideas, and tips with others can make life a little easier.
- See your doctor regularly, no matter how many conflicting demands there are on your time.
- Set aside time just for you. Put yourself on your priority list, and make time to exercise, relax, and enjoy yourself as much as possible.

SHEEHAN'S SYNDROME

Let's just say that you didn't have the easiest pregnancy. After several weeks of warnings from your obstetrician that your delivery could get complicated because of the position of the placenta, the worst came true. Instead of spending your first night as a new mom with your baby, you were alone in your room, getting a blood transfusion to replace the significant amount of blood you lost during the delivery.

Now, six weeks later, you're back at the doctor's office. You don't feel right: You were never able to breastfeed and instead of your breasts filling with milk, they actually managed to shrink. You are exhausted all the time and are parched with thirst. You go through more than two gallons of bottled water a day.

What's wrong?

You may have something called *Sheehan's syndrome*, a condition where your pituitary gland loses its blood supply and can no longer function properly. The pituitary gland is located at the base of your brain. It secretes hormones and regulates a wide variety of your body's activities.

During pregnancy, the pituitary gland increases in size, making it vulnerable to the effects of severe blood loss such as occurs in a postpartum hemorrhage. Without a blood supply, the gland doesn't receive enough oxygen and, depending on how severe it is, will function minimally or not at all.

Is it common?

Sheehan's syndrome is not often seen in the United States today. It is more common in developing countries. But when seen here, it is particularly likely to occur in women who experienced serious blood loss during their pregnancies and/or deliveries.

What are the symptoms?

The symptoms vary depending on the severity of blood loss and ensuing damage to the pituitary gland. The most common symptoms include: low blood pressure, an inability to produce milk and breastfeed, breast shrinkage, low blood sugar, absence of menstrual period, fatigue and weakness, loss of bodily hair in the pubic region and under the arm, and extreme thirst (brought on by a special form of diabetes). All of the symptoms are caused by the pituitary gland's inability to secrete hormones and regulate the body's normal processes.

The symptoms may occur immediately after the delivery or may not manifest until months or years later.

How is Sheehan's syndrome diagnosed?

If a doctor suspects that you have Sheehan's syndrome, she/he will give you a thorough physical exam and ask many questions about your medical history and current symptoms. A number of tests can help with the diagnosis, including blood tests and hormonal assays, stimulation checks of your brain function, and CT and MRI imaging.

How is it treated?

Thankfully, Sheehan's syndrome can be successfully managed and treated with hormone substitution medication. Depending on the extent of damage to the pituitary gland, a person can expect to take lifelong estrogen, progesterone, and adrenal and thyroid hormone supplements. If diagnosed and treated early, patients with this syndrome have an excellent prognosis and life expectancy.

DIABETES

At twenty-six weeks, you went into the lab for a glucose tolerance test. You chugged a pretty nasty-tasting orange drink and sat in the waiting room for what seemed like an eternity. Your name was finally called and a technician took some blood and that was it. Or so you thought. You had all but forgotten about the test when the phone rang a few days later. Your test was positive, you were told, and you needed to come back for a three-hour marathon test. You brought a big, fat novel to read and pitched a tent in the waiting room. You were a little nervous. *Not to worry,* the nurse told you, *most women who test positive the first time get a normal result with the longer test.*

Unfortunately, your test comes out positive again. When they called to tell you your diagnosis of gestational diabetes, you were told to meet with your doctor to get a plan to help you manage your condition.

For the sake not only of your own health but especially of the baby's, your doctor encouraged you to maintain a strict diet-and-exercise routine and showed you how to monitor your blood sugar levels. You strictly adhered to the plan, eating properly and exercising every day. Your efforts paid off and everything turned out okay. You are now at home with a healthy baby.

Six weeks later, you get a reminder card for a follow-up appointment at the doctor's office to make sure your sugar levels are back to normal. You start to get anxious again and worry that the diabetes might not have gone away.

What is gestational diabetes?

Gestational diabetes is a special form of diabetes that manifests during pregnancy. For reasons that are not clear, the body becomes unable to utilize glucose, or sugar, properly and the levels increase in the bloodstream. Typically, this form of diabetes shows up in the middle of the pregnancy, during the fifth or sixth month. Women with gestational diabetes often have larger babies than women without diabetes.

Will the diabetes stick around?

Probably not. Studies have shown that in most cases, gestational diabetes disappears after the baby is born. In a very small percentage of women, the diabetes persists after the baby is born. These women will probably need to be treated by a doctor who can help monitor and manage the condition.

How would you know if you still had diabetes after the baby was born?

The best way to find out is to have another glucose tolerance test at your six-week postpartum visit. This often involves fasting overnight and getting a blood test in the office. Some women with persistent diabetes complain of extreme thirst or frequent urination. But most of the time, the symptoms are nonexistent or so subtle that you wouldn't realize anything was wrong.

What do I need to do if the diabetes is still present after delivery?

Try to maintain the same good habits that helped keep your blood sugar levels in check during your pregnancy. This may be particularly challenging during the postpartum period, which can be a hectic time, to say the least. Skipping meals, lack of sleep, and stress can all put you at risk for low or erratic blood sugar levels. Monitor your levels closely and make the time to keep a written record of all numbers. And be sure to follow up with your doctor at regular intervals. Just because you are caring for another little person doesn't mean you should neglect yourself.

Can you breastfeed if you still have diabetes?

The answer is yes. According to the American Diabetes Association, women with gestational diabetes should be encouraged to breastfeed. Both the mom and baby will reap the benefits. For baby, breastfeeding may protect against certain illnesses later down the road. For Mom, breastfeeding may actually help lower blood sugar levels. Speak with your nurse or lactation consultant for special instructions.

Any tips for preventing low blood sugar levels during breastfeeding?

For all breastfeeding women but especially those with diabetes, drinking enough is vital. Make sure to stay well-hydrated throughout the day. Always have at least one eight-ounce glass of water or other beverage before a breastfeeding session begins. Some doctors recommend having a snack before or during breastfeeding too.

Will you get diabetes with the next pregnancy?

You might. Roughly two-thirds of all women with gestational diabetes are diagnosed with it again in subsequent pregnancies. So you and your doctor should both be on the lookout for gestational diabetes, and if you switch health care practitioners between pregnancies, make sure to alert the new one about your medical history.

Are you at risk for diabetes later in life?

Unfortunately, yes. Women with gestational diabetes have an increased risk of developing type 2 diabetes later in life. The risk goes up if you are obese, lead a sedentary lifestyle, and/or you needed medication to control your diabetes during pregnancy. The good news is that you can lower your chances by eating healthy meals, exercising regularly, and maintaining a proper weight.

P.S. Your child may be at an increased risk for obesity and diabetes later in life. So make sure to serve healthy meals and encourage plenty of exercise. Discuss this issue with your child's pediatrician for additional tips and advice.

3

Your Breastfeeding Self

There are hundreds if not thousands of books available about the virtues of breastfeeding—but this isn't one of them. I am not here to lecture you on the health benefits of breastfeeding, or to make you feel like a total loser if you decide not to do it. (Please note: There are many people out there who are smart and healthy who were bottle-fed as infants.) I am simply here to tell you how to take care of your breasts if you do indeed choose to breastfeed, and how to recognize common problems if they arise. My mission is to address common breastfeeding concerns from a physical and emotional standpoint. So if you are breastfeeding, this chapter's for you.

I'd like to start by sharing my own story. While pregnant with my first child, I read many, many books about breastfeeding. (Thinking back, I can't believe how much free time

I had, but that's another story.) Wanting what was best for my unborn child, and convinced that this was the right choice for both of us, especially from a health standpoint, I was determined to succeed at breastfeeding.

So there I was, headed to the hospital with suitcase in hand, a pregnancy book under one arm, and a breastfeeding book under the other. After a long labor and three hours of pushing, my darling daughter emerged looking adorable, with a red cone head to match my red and exhausted swollen face. Thankfully, we were both fine.

The nurses brought my baby to me that first night and I attempted to breastfeed. I had bookmarked the pages in my childbirth manual and read them many times previously, but I just couldn't follow the directions now that I was holding a real baby; they didn't make any sense. Football hold? Cradle position? Lie down with baby? This was proving to be trickier than my biochemistry class in medical school. My daughter wouldn't open her mouth, even though the book promised she would as soon as the nipple touched it. And was my milk even in yet?

I was exhausted and quickly becoming exasperated, too. Here I was with my new baby and I couldn't even feed her. I fell asleep feeling like a total failure. The next morning, the nurses came to my rescue. They sat with me for over an hour, and my daughter finally latched on before we left. At last, I had the hang of it . . . or so I thought.

Once I got home, she didn't latch on at all. I was so engorged and in so much pain, I didn't know what to do. So I did what many new moms do . . . I called my own mom. And of course, she had the solution. Two hours later, her good friend, whom I will call "Breastfeeder Betty," a woman who would make the La Leche League proud, breezed through the door. She instantly ordered me to show her my breasts. Was she kidding? Apparently not, because she waited until I opened my blouse, then grabbed one sore, enlarged, and engorged breast and squeezed it hard, to show me how to do it. You know when the doctor asks you to rate your pain on the scale from one to ten—this, my friends, was a ten. This was an epidural, painkiller, gimme-anything-you-got ten. But I had just made it through childbirth, and if you can do that, you can do anything. So, I sucked this pain up too, took notes, and believe it or not, started successfully breastfeeding on my own that night. (Betty had gone home, thank you, Lord.)

Over the next few months, I suffered from sore nipples, one of which actually cracked. And several of my friends were having their own problems. One had mastitis, an infection of the breast; another had a plugged duct; and still another couldn't breastfeed at all—she just didn't produce enough milk, and gave up trying after a few weeks. Those of us going back to work struggled with the obvious issues of pumping and storing, supplementing, or giving it up altogether. Breastfeeding turned out to be one of those topics we discussed for hours among ourselves. Who would ever have guessed before having a baby how fascinating we would find it?

FREQUENTLY ASKED QUESTIONS

It's only been two days since I started breastfeeding and my breasts are killing me. Why?

Once your milk starts to come in, and the milk volume quickly increases—which usually occurs sometime during the first week after delivery—your breasts have a tendency to become overfilled, or "engorged," and this can be quite painful. It may take a while for your body to learn how to regulate your milk production and for you to get the hang of breastfeeding. Until then, it is easy for your breasts to become engorged.

Many experts recommend breastfeeding frequently to avoid engorgement. As soon as your breasts start to feel firm, it's important to relieve the pressure. If the baby has been fully fed and is sound asleep, pumping, manually expressing, taking a warm shower, or even just gently massaging your breasts may do the trick.

What is colostrum?

Colostrum is the yellowish-colored liquid your breasts start to secrete right after delivery. It is filled with important nutrients and infection-fighting antibodies. Colostrum secretion continues for about five days, with a gradual transfer to mature milk during the next four weeks.

How do I know if I'm producing enough milk?

Many women, at one point or another, worry that their babies aren't getting enough milk. And who can blame them? It's not that easy figuring out how much the baby has gotten from your breasts, and if the breasts have emptied, or whether the baby is full. It's not like a bottle, where you can see how much the baby has consumed. Here are a few indicators of a well-fed baby:

- If the baby seems satisfied after each meal
- If the baby is steadily gaining weight (but don't freak out if the baby loses some weight in the first week or so. That's to be expected.)
- If you're changing about six to eight wet diapers a day
- If the baby is having more than two stools a day (though this can vary a lot, and the number will usually decrease as time goes on.)

If you don't feel that you are producing enough milk, don't hesitate to contact a nurse, lactation specialist, or your doctor. Until then, you can try to increase the number of feedings a day. Usually, the more often you feed, the more milk you'll produce. But everyone is different and a specialist may be able to offer better advice tailored specifically to you and your baby.

Is my baby affected by what I eat?

Definitely. When you're breastfeeding, it's important to eat a well-balanced meal, and also to notice if certain foods don't seem to agree with your baby. Some women swear that spicy or gassy foods affect their babies; other women don't notice a difference. If it seems to you that your baby is bothered by a certain food, you may want to avoid it. Just make sure to fill your diet with healthy foods.

Caffeine and alcohol can make their way into your breast milk, so it's important to limit these substances while breastfeeding. Certain drugs, including nicotine, can also affect your breast milk. Make sure to speak with your doctor or nurse about any medications you are taking, because they can best advise you about whether these will affect your baby.

Help! I'm a leaky faucet.

I can relate! A few years ago, about five weeks after I had my daughter, I was a bridesmaid at the wedding of one of my best friends. The tag inside my dress read: "Do not get wet!" As we walked down the aisle, I heard a baby cry and sure enough, I started leaking. And we're not talking about a slow leak; I was literally leaking like a faucet. I held my flowers tight to my chest, but when the ceremony was over, there were two large rings on the top of my lavender dress. Needless to say, I wore a T-shirt the rest of the night. And I left the dress in the closet of the hotel when I checked out!

Almost everyone I know has a story like this. Here are a few tips to avoid Niagara Falls at your best friend's wedding:

- Use disposable pads, make sure they are lined up properly, and change them frequently (especially if you're at an event where you can't breastfeed frequently)!
- Try to stop the "let-down" reflex by putting pressure on your chest. Crossing your arms sometimes works; other times, there's little you can do but grin and bear it!
- Try to breastfeed frequently, especially in the beginning as your body is trying to regulate. It's more common

to leak during the first few weeks. So, if you find yourself at an event, unable to breastfeed, don't forget your pump!

NIPPLES

Your nipples are killing you. They're tender and sensitive and you cringe every time the baby latches on. Come to think of it, the mere thought of a baby nursing makes you want to run for the hills!

Why are your nipples so sore?

The most common reason for sore nipples is incorrect positioning of the baby during breastfeeding. You'll want to address this issue as soon as possible because it shouldn't hurt to breastfeed. Make sure the baby's mouth opens widely to fit in the entire nipple and areola area (darkened area around the nipple) when latching on.

Some babies have a harder time with this, so if the baby isn't latched-on properly, take the baby right off the breast and try again. The best way to release the suction is to put a finger in the corner of the baby's mouth between the gums.

You've tried all the positions, but your nipples still hurt. What else can you do?

There are some other things you can try. If one nipple is particularly sore, try nursing with the other one first. Remember, a hungry baby has a very strong suck reflex, especially at the start of the feed. Spare the sore nipple by introducing the other one; by the time the baby gets around to the sore nipple, the suck won't be as robust.

Some studies have shown that breast milk can actually help soothe and heal sore nipples. Try rubbing some on your nipples after you breastfeed and let them air dry. Don't rush to put your bra back on either; give those poor nipples some air.

One nipple is cracked and bleeding; is there anything I can do?

Many women mistakenly think that cracked and bleeding nipples are just part of breastfeeding. But there is a big difference between **sore** nipples, where the skin is *not* broken and **cracked** nipples, where the skin *is* broken. A cracked and/or bleeding nipple is not a normal part of the whole process and needs your prompt attention.

Many experts recommend using lanolin or a similar product on your breasts before and after breastfeeding to prevent problems. Once the skin on the nipple is broken, "moist wound healing"—the use of lanolin or a hydrogel to maintain a moist environment—can help mend the nipple and hasten healing. Ask your doctor, nurse, or lactation consultant for further advice.

Can you still breastfeed if there's blood in the milk?

It is safe to breastfeed your baby if your nipple is bleeding. The blood won't harm her. If you are very uncomfortable, some experts recommend breast shields, which can help ease your pain and let you continue breastfeeding while the breast heals. Continue using the lanolin or other wound-healing products until you feel better.

PLUGGED DUCT(S)

There's something hard in your areola (the darker area around the nipple) and you're starting to worry. It feels like a lump and it hurts when you push on it. There's an area of redness near the spot and the pain seems to come and go.

Is it a tumor?

Lumps in the breast tend to elicit fear in most women, no matter what their age. But this one sounds more like a plugged duct. Occasionally a milk duct, one of the tube-shaped passageways that carries milk to your nipple, can get blocked. The result: a painful, hard lump in the breast.

What causes it?

Several things can cause a plugged duct, but the most common is inadequate emptying of the breast during a feed. Rushed feedings, a defective breast pump, or a baby falling asleep on the job can all contribute to the inability of the breast to fully empty. Other causes of plugged ducts include: stress, illness, exhaustion, and a tight bra. Sometimes, the underlying reason for a plugged duct cannot be determined.

What can you do about it?

You should try to unplug the area as soon as possible because if you don't address the problem, the duct could get infected. Here are some suggestions:

- Put the baby on the affected side first. As I mentioned before, a hungry baby has a very strong suck reflex and will most likely empty the affected breast, and possibly dislodge the plug.
- Do it yourself. You can massage the affected breast (even if it hurts) and try to express extra milk and loosen the plug.
- Try warm soaks. Some experts recommend soaking the breast in warm water or applying moist, warm washcloths to the area.

If none of these work, speak with your doctor or nurse for more suggestions.

Not only do you have a plugged duct, but you have a fever and feel like you have the flu.

You might have a breast infection. Don't ignore your symptoms, especially if the pain and redness are increasing and if you have a fever. It would be wise to seek medical attention because you might need a prescription.

Are there any ways to prevent plugged ducts from happening?

There are a few things you can do to lower your chances of getting a plugged duct. Try to empty each breast when you are nursing. If your baby tends to snooze, wake him/her up and try to finish the feed, if possible. Avoid tight bras at all costs. Not only are they uncomfortable, but they can cause problems. Many maternity stores have attendants who can help fit you properly. When in doubt, ask for help.

But remember, plugged ducts can sometimes occur without reason. So be aware of the warning signs and make sure to address the problem, if it occurs.

MASTITIS

You've been breastfeeding for almost six weeks, when you notice that one of your breasts is red, swollen, and painful. When you touch it, it feels warm. You've been feeling really run-down and tired, but you just assumed it was from all those middle-of-the-night feeding sessions. But now that your breast hurts, you wonder if it's more than just normal fatigue.

Is something else wrong?

Very likely. You may have mastitis, which literally means an inflammation of the breast. Most often, it occurs within the first three months of breastfeeding. The breast is usually red, swollen, painful, and warm to the touch. In the vast majority of cases, mastitis involves only one breast, not both.

Why does it happen?

Mastitis can occur when bacteria make their way into the breast, usually through a milk duct or a break in the skin of the nipple. Remember, your baby's mouth has bacteria in it, so if you have cracked or sore nipples, your risk of infection goes up! Your risk of mastitis can also increase if you've had it before, if you have plugged ducts, or if you use only one position to breastfeed the baby.

What are the most common signs of mastitis?

Aside from redness, swelling, and pain, some women also experience flu-like symptoms, exhaustion, fever (usually 101 degrees or higher), and pain or burning while breastfeeding.

If you feel run-down or achy, have a fever and/or chills, it is likely that the breast has become infected. Some women get these symptoms before the breast becomes swollen and red. It's important to go see the doctor because you may need a prescription for antibiotics in order to clear up the infection.

Do you definitely need antibiotics?

Not necessarily. It is possible to have painful and swollen breasts without an infection, especially if you have no fever. But you should see the doctor anyway, because it's usually tricky to figure out whether your breast has become infected. The doctor will best be able to guide you and offer treatment, if required.

Will mastitis go away on its own if you don't treat it?

No! Ignoring the symptoms of mastitis will not make it go away. In fact, you may be putting yourself at risk for something even more serious called an abscess. An abscess is a collection of pus and can result if the infection is not treated properly. This usually requires surgical intervention and drainage—something you definitely do not want to deal with. So make sure to seek help if you suspect that you have an infection.

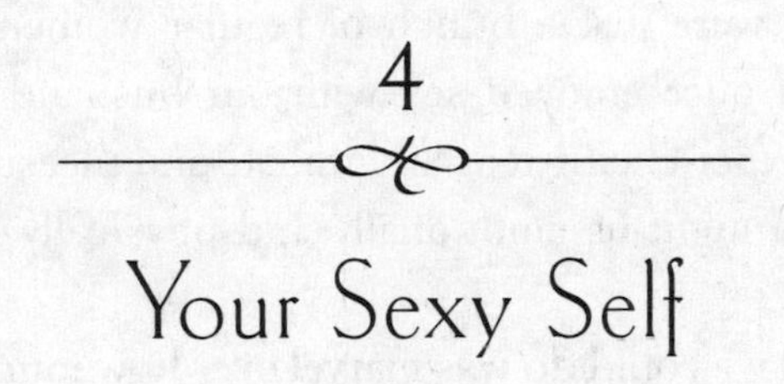

4

Your Sexy Self

Want to stir up some interesting reactions? Walk into a room filled with new moms and ask this simple question: How's your sex life now?

This seemingly harmless question can evoke some strong reactions from some pretty exhausted women who are likely to rank sex at the very bottom of the list of things they want to do after having a baby. An equally strong reaction comes from the select (few) women jumping right back into the sack after having a baby.

So what is it about sex after pregnancy that gets new moms going? After all, it was sex that got us here in the first place. For starters, it's the fact that our sex lives—scratch that, our entire lives—have changed dramatically, especially if this is baby number one. In my new moms group, many of the conversations that attempted to address other aspects of our lives inevitably ended up in an exchange about sex—or the lack of sex. And it wasn't like we had once been sexaholics; we were just a bunch of regular women, most of whom had once enjoyed sex with our husbands and our partners, experiencing it as an intimate and pleasurable act, one that brought us emotionally and physically closer together.

Now all we could do was marvel over how much havoc a small baby could wreak on something that had once been so natural and spontaneous.

After the baby, we all agreed, sex was different. Our bodies had just gone through a miraculous process, but one that left behind enough bruises and scars to make the very thought of sex send shivers of dread down some of our spines. And we were exhausted, not just from the delivery, but from the endless sleepless nights that ensued. Some of our husbands were feeling left out, marginalized, as the baby became our central focus. Sex had never seemed so important to them—or so unimportant to us. The more they longed to feel close and connected, the more we longed to . . . well, really, just get some sleep!

Depending on what type of delivery we had and what complications there were, if any, there were different issues to face. In general, for vaginal deliveries, if a woman has an episiotomy or tear during her delivery, her recovery time may be longer, especially if the laceration is deep. It can take weeks or even months for the pain to subside completely.

My own war story, which I share only to convince you that I feel your pain, involved a fairly extensive episiotomy with my first child because she was occiput posterior, meaning she was delivered sunny-side up, with her face looking at the ceiling, instead of the more common other way around. After having back labor for what seemed like an eternity, I had pushed for more than two additional hours. So I was very sore indeed in the aftermath (though "sore" is really an understatement). When my obstetrician told me at my six-week appointment that I could now have sex, I told her that she must be on drugs. It wasn't until several months later that I even considered taking her up on her suggestion.

One of my friends, however, had a planned Cesarean section which went quite smoothly. She was in pain for about two weeks after the delivery and then quickly started to feel much better. At her six-week appointment, she was told that she could have sex again. And so she did, and never looked back.

Every woman I have spoken to had different issues, different timetables, and different thoughts on the subject at hand. For many postpartum women, there are a variety of obstacles to overcome including: low sex drive, wounds that are still healing, painful intercourse, exhaustion, fluctuating hormone levels, lack of vaginal lubrication, and decreased sense of attractiveness, to name just a few. For other women, there seem to be no issues at all. So, there is no one answer to when to have sex, how to have sex, or how much sex to have after you have a baby. You just need to listen to your body, your mind, and your heart.

BODY IMAGE PROBLEMS

After the baby comes, it's only a matter of time before most women declare that they want their old bodies back. It's almost as if a little alien had been occupying the body, stretching it and contorting it in all different directions. Now that the alien has vacated, it's time for women to reclaim what is rightfully theirs—their looks, their sexuality, their energy and ease of movement.

However, the postpartum period isn't the sexiest-looking time, which can be upsetting, especially for women who place a high value on their appearance. And it's probably not the sexiest-*feeling* time in a woman's life either, to say the least. During pregnancy, some women feel super sexy and enjoy a healthy and active sex life. Other women don't feel sexy at all. But regardless of the state of mind women are in during those nine months, most will agree that during the time immediately after the baby comes and for several weeks to months later, the idea of sex is somewhere between a low priority and a nightmare. Even if they are not in a state of pain or exhaustion, they're self-conscious about how their bodies now look.

But aren't we too hard on ourselves? Take a minute and think about the incredible thing your body has just done, and the load it had to carry to do it. Besides the baby, you've been carrying the weight of the placenta, amniotic fluid, retained water, increased blood supply, distended uterus, engorged breasts, and maternal fat stores—a total of an extra twenty-five to thirty-five pounds on average. Even though much of that weight came off as soon as you delivered, you may not realize that the additional fat that got deposited and stored throughout the pregnancy is not going to disappear along with the weight of the baby, the placenta, and all those fluids. This extra fat is there to provide energy for the mother during and after the pregnancy, when she breastfeeds.

Unfortunately, once these cells are deposited, they're not going anywhere. You can't exercise them away. You can make them smaller by getting regular exercise and eating healthily, but get used to them because they're here to stay. So, cut yourself some slack! It may take months on end to shrink those annoying cells down to size.

And it's not just the fat cells doing a number on your "new" body. For starters, your breasts are larger than normal with huge nipples, especially if you're breastfeeding. Your beautifully taut pregnant belly has been turned into a wasteland of extra, flabby skin. Depending on how you delivered, you may have a variety of wounds and scars that are just beginning to heal and in the meantime looking quite horrifying.

The take-home message: Give yourself time—time to heal, time to shed those pounds slowly and steadily. The last thing you need to do right now is stress about your body. But there are strategies for dealing with many of the sex-related issues that arise during this challenging period, some of which will help you to develop the patience you need to endure it, and some of which may help you shorten it. So read on and take heart.

I hate my body and I'm too self-conscious to get it on with my husband.

You are definitely not alone. Many women have problems accepting their post-baby bodies. Some stress over the stretch marks, scars, and extra pounds; others fear that their partners won't view their bodies in the same way they did before the baby came. One mother told me that her husband couldn't watch her breastfeed because he didn't want to picture her breasts in a nonsexual way!

No matter what issue you may be grappling with, accepting your postpartum body can be tough. Most women I spoke with found the adjustment to their new postpartum shape as difficult as dealing with the changes of pregnancy. Loose, flabby skin has replaced that rounded, tight belly, and it just doesn't want to go away! Many women feel that there is no excuse for the extra pounds after the baby comes. They want their pre-pregnancy bodies back pronto and can end up feeling frustrated and self-conscious if it doesn't happen right away.

As a result, some women will pass up intimate contact with their partners in an attempt to avoid exposing their "undesirable bodies." Others suffer from a reduced sex drive based on feelings of embarrassment and/or fear of rejection. For most women, these feelings pass as they get back into shape.

Here are a few tips for dealing with your post-pregnancy body and keeping the spark alive:

- Review your expectations. If you were under the impression that you'd slip right back into your hippest pair of jeans right after the baby was born, you may need to accept that for most women, this just isn't realistic. Sure, there are the lucky few who can be seen lounging poolside in sexy bikinis three or four weeks post-baby, but if you're reading this, you are probably not among them.

  Remember, it takes time and effort to get that body back. And a few extra pounds, plus a stretch mark or three (and a varicose vein), shouldn't stop you from getting it on with your partner, especially if you're in the mood. Some of these changes will fade or disappear altogether, but others may be here to stay, so you'll have to get used to them. Chances are your partner will be so excited to get a little action, he won't care about the changes you're obsessing about.

- Give yourself a break. You've just been through a tremendous event that has taken an inevitable toll on your body. You should feel beautiful and proud, not embarrassed or self-conscious. That body of yours is a magnificent organism which has just produced a baby. What a great gift it has given you. Love yourself from the inside out, and give yourself the time and emotional space to gradually get back into shape.
- Keep in mind: Sex doesn't necessarily correlate with pounds. Among my mommy friends, the woman with the most active sex life was the one who was the last to lose her extra pounds.
- Dim the lights. As basic as this tip sounds, the advice can go a long way. Turning down the lights can actually make you feel more comfortable. You won't need to worry that your partner is taking notice of all of your imperfections. You can just focus on making each other feel desired! To make it more romantic, light a scented candle and play some mood music.
- If you're breastfeeding, stop worrying about leakage. Some women worry that their breasts will leak during sexual activity—so much that the anxiety gets in the way of their libido. Wearing a nursing bra with pads

can do the trick, both because it solves the problem and because it reduces anxiety about the problem.

LOW SEX DRIVE

He looks at you across the dinner table on your first night out since the baby was born. He's flirting, you think, but you hardly notice because you've been secretly checking your watch under the table, counting the minutes until you can get home to make sure your babysitter hasn't dropped the baby.

He reaches for your hand; you're still thinking about the baby. You hear something in the background which sounds like a baby and your breasts fill up with milk. He tells you how much he loves you and you start to leak. He is definitely trying to set the stage for a romantic and intimate evening and you, on the other hand, have to excuse yourself to change your breast pad in the bathroom.

How can he think about sex when sex is the furthest thing from your mind? You haven't thought about sex for, well, it's been about four months. Last night, he told you that he misses being with you. You start to feel bad. But then you check your watch again; only fifteen more minutes, you think, and then you can go home and be with the baby.

How come you're not in the mood (at all)?

There are so many explanations for why new moms aren't in the mood to have sex after the baby comes. A low sex drive can be frustrating for both you and your partner.

But don't despair; it's a normal part of the picture. Reasons for a decreased libido include:

- Fluctuating hormone levels. After the baby is born, estrogen and progesterone levels drop, which can contribute to a decrease in your sex drive. If you are breastfeeding, a hormone called prolactin becomes elevated, which can further suppress the other hormone levels, and with them, your sexual desire. It can take months for your hormone levels to go back to their pre-pregnancy levels.
- Fatigue. I don't need to tell you that new moms frequently suffer from exhaustion. But fatigue and exhaustion can wreak more havoc on your body than you may realize. Studies have shown that disrupted sleep, night after night, can contribute to stress, moodiness, poor decision-making, a decreased immune response, and lowered sex drive.
- Concern about the way your body looks. As discussed above, many women are self-conscious about the changes in their bodies during the postpartum period and anxious about whether their partners will still find their bodies attractive. While these feelings are normal, they can get in the way of the desire to be intimate with your partner.
- Pain. Depending on the type of delivery you experienced, you may have incisions that have not yet healed and are still quite painful. Even if there is no episiotomy or Cesarean scar, the perineum, or area between the vaginal and rectal openings, has been stretched

(beyond belief) and is most likely pretty sore. For many women, the thought of putting anything even close to that area can evoke fear and anxiety, which in turn can dramatically lessen sexual desire.

- Lack of vaginal lubrication. In breastfeeding women, elevated prolactin levels and lowered estrogen and progesterone levels can result in vaginal dryness. Without proper lubrication, sex can hurt, and as a result, women may steer away from relations with their partners, especially while breastfeeding.

It's been six weeks and I'm definitely not ready to have sex. Is something wrong with me? Are most women ready at this point?

No, nothing is wrong with you. Some women just take longer than others to be ready. I can't stress enough how individualized this all is. The decision to have sex after the baby comes is definitely not a one-size-fits-all milestone. Everyone is different. I knew women who had sex again right at the six-week mark and others who didn't have sex until the baby's first birthday!

Doctors recommend waiting six weeks because it gives the body a chance to heal. At this point, for most women, postpartum bleeding will have stopped, tears, sutures, and lacerations will be healed, and the cervix will have closed. But that doesn't necessarily mean you feel ready. Many women complain of pain and soreness well after the six-week mark. Other women deal with some of the issues we've already discussed. The decision to resume relations with your partner is entirely up to you. Don't let the six-week timeline—or pressure from your partner—dictate your decision; you need to feel comfortable, both mentally and physically.

Help! I'm just too tired to have sex.

Join the club! The new mom's club, that is. Almost every new mother complains of fatigue and exhaustion, especially in the first three months of the baby's life. Fatigue tops the list of reasons that women aren't in the mood for sex in the postpartum period.

Battling exhaustion can be a feat for any new mother, especially if you're only sleeping two- to three-hour stretches at a time. Sleep deprivation not only robs you of your libido, it can take a toll on other aspects of your life, including your emotional well-being.

The good news is: The newborn sleep schedule doesn't last forever! The baby will most likely start to sleep for longer stretches of time into the second and third months of life. Of course, this can vary quite a bit. Some babies sleep for long stretches right away, while others catnap for months on end.

The important thing is that you get enough rest, or at least as much as you can. Studies have shown that sleeping for even four-hour stretches at a time can ease the symptoms of sleep deprivation and help keep your sinking libido from going under.

Here are some tips to maximize your sleep during the newborn haze—that crazy time period before you and the baby get into a good sleep schedule. Feeling well-rested will definitely help keep your sex drive alive:

- Try to sleep when the baby does. You've definitely heard this before, but when that baby goes in for a nap, you need to as well. Even if the baby goes down for less than an hour, lie down and sleep. Naps can recharge you in more ways than one. Don't underestimate the power of a nap when it comes to getting your groove on.

  A note to those of us who can't sleep: For some women, sleeping when the baby does can be a real challenge. With my first child, I could never sleep when she took a nap. My mind was racing. What if she woke up and I didn't hear her? The monitor used to keep me awake, as I jumped up the second I heard a gurgle or sigh. I was also so anxious about being a good mother that when I couldn't sleep I made mental lists of everything I needed to do and read articles on being a parent while she slept. Trying to sleep when the baby slept caused me more anxiety than it was worth. I became stressed thinking, *Why can't I sleep?*

  With my second child, I would collapse the minute he went down for a nap without giving it another thought. Why the difference? It was a "been there, done that" approach. I knew that my son would be okay in the crib even if I wasn't there the second he woke up. Oftentimes, he'd play for a few minutes by himself before I entered the room. And I didn't bother to use the monitor, because I knew I would hear him as soon as he started to cry. Plus, I no longer needed to steal time from sleeping to read all those parenting articles because I had much more confidence in myself as a parent.

So, my advice is, try to turn your mind off while the baby is sleeping. The more relaxed you are, the more likely you'll be able to doze off. And don't stress if you can't sleep. Just use the time to do some deep breathing and stretch out, with your feet up! The more relaxed and rested you are, the more intact your libido and your mind will be.

- Forget the chores. This may be the single best piece of advice I received from my friends who had children before me, especially because I love to multitask. Whatever you do, do NOT worry about the house, house guests, in-laws, the dog, or the dishes when you are exhausted. They can all wait, including your in-laws. The period following the birth of your child can be stressful. Adjusting to a new life with a baby, compounded by dealing with a blunted libido and no sleep, is enough to put anyone over the edge. Take the phone off the hook and throw out your to-do list for now. Rest—you need it and you deserve it!

- Eat well-balanced meals. Do I sound like your mom? If so, we both have a point. Many new moms are so busy, they fail to make time for meals, opting instead to skip meals and fill up on less-than-nutritious snacks. Other moms who are focused on shedding those postpartum pounds begin to diet right away. Skipping meals, snacking, and dieting are all poor choices during this time period.

  Eating healthy meals is vital for you right now. Food provides energy and you need as much energy as you can get. Unhealthy snacks with empty calories will provide you with a short surge of energy, but they're unlikely to sustain you throughout the day. Make sure to eat three healthy meals a day and stick to nutritious snacks including yogurt, whole-grain crackers, fresh fruits, and vegetables. Cut snacks up and keep them in the refrigerator. If you have the urge for junk food (and we all do!), try to satisfy your cravings with something tasty but healthy: low-fat frozen yogurt or sorbet, pretzels, or peanut butter on rice cakes. Remember, fatigue can destroy your libido, and addressing the problem may be as easy as changing your eating habits.

- Drink plenty of fluids. Dehydration can contribute to fatigue in a big way. New moms may get easily dehydrated, especially if they're breastfeeding. One of my friends ended up in the emergency room while she was breastfeeding because she failed to drink enough fluid during the day. Stay hydrated and make sure to drink at least eight to ten glasses of water a day.

  Note: If you are overly exhausted and the feeling seems to persist even when you catch up on sleep, you may have anemia. (See the section on anemia, p. 33.) Other symptoms include pale skin, racing heart, dizziness, and shortness of breath. If you think you have anemia, you should speak to a health care professional.

BREASTFEEDING AND SEX

Studies have shown that breastfeeding can negatively impact a woman's sex life, but this isn't true for everyone. I've spoken to many women who enjoyed a healthy sex life while breastfeeding, so again, it all depends on the person. There's no doubt, however, that breastfeeding does pose some challenges to your sex life, and for women who decide to breastfeed for a prolonged period of time, overcoming these obstacles can become a real hurdle. Here are some of the problems breastfeeding women encounter, and suggestions on how to deal with them.

- Decrease in vaginal lubrication, because of hormone suppression. This can easily be overcome by using a water-based lubricant. It's important to use a water-based lubricant because oil-based lubricants can cause condoms to deteriorate and place you at risk for another pregnancy.
- Lack of sensation in the breasts. Some women complain that their breasts have become less responsive to touch because of all the action they are getting from the baby! Daily feedings can toughen up the nipples, making them less likely to become sexually aroused. If this is the case for you, let your partner know that laying off the breasts for a while may be a good way to go. Using other erogenous zones like the mouth, ears, back of the neck, feet, wrists, or inner thighs may do the trick.
- Leaking breasts. Breast stimulation during foreplay and orgasm can cause the breasts to leak milk. Some women feel embarrassed by this or worry that their partners might feel awkward. Wearing a nursing bra during sexual activity can alleviate the worry and the problem. This issue tends to resolve for women who breastfeed for extended time periods.

- Just not in the mood. One study revealed that breastfeeding women who reported reduced interest in sex had lower levels of androgens, sex hormones produced by the ovaries and adrenal glands in women. If this is happening to you, it can be quite frustrating for you and your partner. Open communication is the key to a healthy relationship. If you have a low sex drive and this feeling persists for an extended period of time, your partner may begin to feel rejected. That's why it is so important to share all of your feelings with your partner. It may also be important to inform your partner about the effects breastfeeding can have on your libido. This knowledge may help the situation.

As far as your sex life goes, you may need to get creative. There are ways to feel close that don't involve sexual intercourse. Spend time together without the baby. Hold hands, cuddle in bed or take a bath together. Kissing and snuggling can make you feel very close. Until you are ready to have sex, look for ways to express affection. Your hormone levels and your libido will most likely return to normal after you stop breastfeeding.

PHYSICAL ROADBLOCKS TO SEX

Fear and Pain

So maybe you're actually in the mood, but the thought of having sex makes you cringe because your body really hurts. It's no surprise that you're in pain: Think about it—just like an Olympic athlete, you've trained for nine months and performed an amazing physical feat that has left your body totally exhausted. Your body is spent: Every muscle aches, every ligament hurts, and you're sore in more places than you care to mention. But you did it! And your gold medal is that beautiful baby. You want to celebrate with your partner, but having sex is out of the question. And it's not because you aren't in the right frame of mind, it's because your body just can't.

If you are in pain, you're certainly not alone. Most women are pretty sore for at least a few weeks after the delivery. Vaginal, rectal, and back pain are all common complaints. But depending on your course of labor and the type of delivery you've had, you may experience some particularly challenging physical roadblocks to intimacy.

Vaginal Deliveries

Recovery time from a vaginal delivery is usually shorter than the recovery time from a Cesarean section. But sometimes it can take a while, especially if you've experienced any lacerations or tears.

The perineum, or the region between the vagina and rectum, is vulnerable to tearing during delivery. Some studies show that women are more likely to tear during their first vaginal delivery, probably because this is the first time the area has been stretched to that degree. But whether it's your first or your tenth, delivery technique can make a huge difference. One study revealed that if normal, spontaneous vaginal deliveries are unrushed and occur in a controlled setting with a nurse, doctor, or midwife guiding the pushing process, there is a lower risk of obstetrical trauma. Many health experts recommend perineal massage in the weeks prior to delivery as a way to lower the chances of tearing. Unfortunately, some women experience tears despite their own best efforts and the efforts of their health care professional.

Tears and Lacerations

Tears and lacerations vary in severity and are classified accordingly:

- **First-degree tears** are surface tears that involve the skin of the perineum and the vaginal connective tissue, usually near the vaginal opening. No muscles are involved. Healing time for first-degree tears is rapid, and women usually experience little discomfort. Stitches may or may not be required.
- **Second-degree tears** are deeper tears that involve the skin, connective tissue, and underlying muscles. Second-degree tears almost always require stitches, and healing time can vary. Most often, the stitches will dissolve on their own. Some women report feeling fine in a matter of weeks, others complain of experiencing pain for longer periods of time.
- **Third-degree tears** are more severe and involve the skin, connective tissue, and the external anal sphincter muscle, the muscle that you can squeeze to stop yourself from going to the bathroom.
- **Fourth-degree tears** are the most severe and can involve a tear through both the internal and external anal

sphincter muscles and lining of the bowel. These tears often result in the loss of anal sphincter control, as well as fecal urgency and/or incontinence.

While third- and fourth-degree perineal tears are not common, they can happen to anyone. There are a few risk factors which may increase the chances:

- Larger babies
- Occiput posterior deliveries (baby is sunny-side up, or delivered faceup, instead of facedown)
- Nulliparity (delivery of first babies)
- Extended second stage of labor, or if the pushing stage lasts longer than an hour
- Midline episiotomies—unfortunately, some women end up tearing further than the controlled incision
- Forceps delivery

Third- and fourth-degree lacerations can be extremely painful and may interfere with all sorts of activities, including intercourse, for quite some time after delivery. Many women find going to the bathroom, especially having a bowel movement, a huge challenge. One woman with a third-degree tear told me that having bowel movements after her delivery was worse than the actual delivery itself.

The pain can persist for months after the baby arrives. A thorough follow-up is very important, so make sure that you see your health care professional several times after the delivery. Your doctor should examine the area and make sure the anorectal area is functioning properly. For many women, the pain and discomfort will subside within a few months and normal activities, including sex, can be resumed.

Some moms experience uncontrollable gas and/or fecal incontinence down the line. These problems should be brought to the attention of your physician immediately. In some cases, additional treatment may be necessary.

Episiotomies

An episiotomy is a controlled surgical incision made in the perineal area (between the vagina and rectum), prior to the delivery. In the past, the episiotomy was used routinely in order to lower the risk of vaginal tears during deliveries. But because newer studies have shown that these routine episiotomies have no real benefit for the mother, and may actually worsen the outcome and prolong healing time, episiotomies are becoming less common. In fact, several studies reveal that more severe lacerations were associated with the occurrence of an episiotomy.

Despite the new research about episiotomies, some women still get them. And it's certainly true that in some cases, an episiotomy may be necessary, especially if the baby presents in an unusual position or is overly large; it may also be necessary if the doctor needs to speed up the delivery for health or medical reasons pertaining to the mom and/or the baby.

Recovery from an episiotomy is a lot like the recovery from a tear; it all depends on the extent of the cut or laceration. For most women, the pain and tenderness will subside significantly in one to two months. If a woman experiences a serious tear in addition to the surgical incision, recovery time may be prolonged.

C-section

The recovery from a Cesarean section, or the delivery of a baby through an abdominal incision, varies from woman to woman. In general, recovery time tends to be longer than the time it takes to recover from a normal, vaginal delivery, unless, of course, a severe tear or laceration is involved.

Right off the bat, the incision site will most likely be sore, although some women report that their incision feels numb and tingly. The pain will gradually subside and the numbness should lessen as well (although I've spoken to a few women who never fully regained total sensation in that area). Many women also complain of itchiness around the scar during the healing process. If the itchiness becomes intolerable, speak with your health care provider for options. Some doctors will recommend soothing creams, but others do not, so it's important to get his/her opinion.

Some women who have had a C-section complain of cramps caused by the buildup of gas in the abdomen after surgery. Walking around or light exercise can help. This will usually go away within the first few days post-surgery, but it can linger, especially if you are not moving at all. Speak with your health care professional if it becomes a problem.

Don't be shocked by the way the incision looks! For many women, seeing a dark red scar on the abdomen can be upsetting. But remember, it fades with time (and will likely look a whole lot better in six to eight weeks) and most doctors make the incision low enough that your pubic hair will eventually cover it.

Certain activities may be difficult right after a C-section; even coughing, sneezing, and laughing can be uncomfortable.

Lifting anything heavy is out of the question, and it will be a while before you can have sex again. You also may need to wait to drive a car, especially if you experience pain buckling your seat belt or getting in and out of the car. Getting up and moving are important parts of the healing process, but you shouldn't expect to run a marathon.

Here's a good piece of advice: Don't overdo it! Oftentimes, women don't seem to realize that they have just had *major* abdominal surgery and they feel frustrated that they are unable to move around freely or lift heavy things. One woman I spoke to complained that the stairs in her house posed a major challenge. Another woman was upset that she was in too much pain to be able to cook for her older child. It normally takes an average of six to eight weeks to recover completely from a Cesarean, and for some women it can take several months.

Here are a few more tips to help speed your recovery from a C-section:

- Accept help. As simple as it sounds, it can make a world of difference. Many women are used to doing everything themselves. But this is not the time to be superwoman. Husbands, siblings, parents, friends, and even in-laws make great helpers. If they offer, take them up on it!
- Take it nice and slowly. Many women feel okay by that six-to-eight-week mark, but if you're not among them, don't do anything that makes you uncomfortable. Overexerting yourself can actually prolong the healing process.

- Don't neglect your bowels. If you're taking pain medications, be aware that certain types can cause constipation, which in itself can become a serious problem. Make sure that your bowel movements are regular, and if this starts to become an issue, speak with your health care provider. Stool softeners and laxatives might be necessary.
- Accept the mess. With tons of foot traffic through your home and visits from your extended family, your house may get messy. But you're recovering, so leave it. This is a great opportunity to ask your mother-in-law to help clean up. Even if the mess causes you stress, it's better to leave it for someone else to handle than for you to overexert yourself. Believe me, there will be many messes in the future you can dirty your hands with!

Once I think I may be ready, do you have any advice for reviving my love life with a maximum of pleasure and a minimum of pain?

The best advice is to wait until you are pain-free, as well as comfortable with the idea of having sex again. If not, your fear and anxiety about whether sex will hurt will not make for an enjoyable evening for either you or your partner; those feelings can also wreak havoc on your libido.

Remember, the first few times that you have sex, it may feel strange. You will likely feel a little tender or tight, especially if you've had stitches. Once you are aroused, these feelings will subside.

Here are some other tips to help ease the pain during the first few times:

- Talk to your partner about your fears and concerns. A good heart-to-heart chat can alleviate your partner's anxieties as well as your own.
- Take it slow, particularly the first few times. Even if you aren't in much pain, the anticipation can make your muscles tense, which can magnify whatever pain you may be experiencing. Incorporate foreplay as much as possible; the more stimulated you are, the more enjoyable the experience will be.
- Use a water-based lubricant. This can minimize both friction and pain.
- Be on top. I definitely recommend having sex on top for a while after your delivery. This way, you can control the speed and extent of penetration. The missionary position is not ideal if you are experiencing any pain.
- Try to relax as much as possible. Too many couples invest too much emotional capital in their first act of sex after the delivery. Making it a big symbolic event can backfire and have negative effects on both you and your partner. If that first time doesn't work as well as you expected, then try, try again!

If your pain persists long after the delivery, you may want to see your doctor. There are a myriad of different reasons for pain during intercourse, and a health care provider can help uncover the reason for your discomfort.

Remember . . .

No matter what type of delivery you have had, the initial sexual encounter after the baby comes can be challenging from both a physical and psychological standpoint. Open and honest communication between partners is crucial and can alleviate many of the emotional issues that may arise.

Having sexual intercourse before you are physically ready can be quite painful. It is very important to wait until the postnatal, six-week checkup before having sexual intercourse. And many women end up waiting longer. For most people, it's just a matter of time (weeks to a few months) before they can resume a satisfying and enjoyable sex life again. For others, it can take a while longer. If you are experiencing persistent pain or discomfort for months on end, a visit to the doctor can help get you back on track, so to speak!

5

Your Mindful Self

Ever since you became pregnant, your hormone levels have been totally out of whack and your mood has been as up and down as they are. You've been happy, sad, weepy, anxious, joyful, and scared—sometimes all at once. You've cycled through so many different emotions you can't believe they haven't taken you away in a straitjacket. And when the baby came, you expected it all to stop.

So why hasn't it?

Right after birth, your hormones haven't really settled down yet. In fact, they're on what some would describe as a roller-coaster ride from hell. And during the days, weeks, or sometimes months it takes for your hormone levels to return to normal, your mood may pay the price. Add to your hormone storm the stress of being a new parent, fatigue, lack of sleep, and no sex, and your partner may want a one-way ticket to Guam.

After the baby comes, some lucky women (and their partners) escape the emotional landslide, but for a significant number of women, the postpartum period can pose some hefty psychological challenges. Many women experience mood swings. In fact, a multitude of research studies conclude that roughly fifty to eighty percent of women live through extreme fluctuations in mood and temperament in the period after they have a baby. Some women feel depressed, others have a hard time concentrating or sleeping well, while others feel overwhelmed or anxious; some women go through all of these emotions. Hormones aside, this shouldn't be so surprising. After all, having a baby is one of the greatest life-altering experiences you (and your partner) will ever have. But few women take the time to come to grips with their own emotions.

Like many other women, when my first baby came I did not put my mental well-being at the top of my list of concerns. *Me who?* I used to joke when my mom called and asked me how I was. I just tried to ignore the wild fluctuations of mood and relegate them to the bottom of my priority list, hoping they would pass. After all, who has time to deal with one's own needs once there's a baby in the house? I've spoken to women who complain that they can't even find time to take a shower. And I know the feeling well because I used to take my daughter, strapped in a car seat, into the bathroom every time I showered. Peeking out through the steamy fog in the bathroom every minute or so to make sure she was still okay, I couldn't help but think how symbolic the entire scene was. My head was in a fog—literally and figuratively.

Luckily, my mood swings did eventually even out. But for some women, intense and sometimes difficult feelings linger for months and months. Learning to distinguish feelings that are a "normal" part of early motherhood from feelings that may require further help and attention is very important.

The scope of psychological issues facing new moms varies from person to person. Some women experience mild mood swings, while others go through a serious, clinical depression. The truth is, your emotional well-being can truly dictate how well you approach and handle the challenges of motherhood.

Sorting out your own feelings and recognizing when it is time to go for help is one of the ways you can take good care of yourself—and your baby. The sections that follow will help you understand whether your feelings are getting in the way of your ability to function, and how to go about getting the help you need if they are.

BABY BLUES

You've been so excited for the baby to come, and now that she's here, all you can do is cry! You're not sure what's wrong and your husband is at a loss too. You literally begged him to stay home from work this morning because you're not sure if you can really do this alone. Just thinking about taking care of the baby by yourself makes you really anxious. Your husband calls from work and you snap at him and then you cry. Watching a commercial for cotton underwear makes you cry too. You're not sure what's wrong because you've never been like this before.

What are the baby blues?

If you're a new mom, you've probably heard of the "baby blues," sometimes referred to as "postpartum blues." This term, used to describe the emotional ups and downs of the initial time period after the birth of the baby, is a normal part of early motherhood for many, many women.

The symptoms vary from person to person. Most often, a woman with the "baby blues" experiences:

- irritability
- sadness
- frequent episodes of crying
- mood swings
- anxiety or feelings of being overwhelmed
- a feeling of being incompetent or unable to take care of the baby
- confusion
- changes in appetite and sleeping patterns

The "baby blues" usually peak within the first week of delivery, and the symptoms generally subside over the next few days to weeks. Some women complain that their symptoms are on and off for several weeks after delivery; others experience a peak in symptoms right after they stop breastfeeding.

Is it common?

Yes. Most new moms will experience periods of mood swings, sadness, weepiness, and confusion during the first few weeks after delivery. Some studies reveal as many as eighty percent of women will go through some form of the "baby blues" in the early period following the birth of the baby.

What brings on the "baby blues"?

There's no right answer to that question because what causes the "baby blues" can vary from person to person. But fluctuating hormone levels seem to play a prominent role for many women. After the baby is born, estrogen and progesterone levels drop. Since these hormones are known to regulate chemicals in the brain that influence mood, it's not surprising that when the hormone levels drop, your emotions are affected.

But hormones aren't the only player. In fact, some studies have explored feelings of sadness and mood swings in new dads, which obviously have little to do with a drop in female hormones. Another possible cause of the "baby blues" is feeling overwhelmed with a new sense of responsibility. Many women feel protected and taken care of in the hospital by the doctors, nurses, and family members. But when a new mom returns home, the enormity of her responsibility may become apparent in a way she might not have recognized while she was still in the hospital. She may feel temporarily overwhelmed, nervous, sad, and/or isolated.

Yet another possible cause of the "baby blues" is what some experts call a "mourning period." Some women mourn the "loss" of their former life, their independence and autonomy, or their freedom. Others actually mourn the end of the pregnancy itself, having become accustomed to carrying a baby around for nine months. While there's a lack of scientific evidence in this department, it is quite clear that having a baby evokes strong feelings in many women.

And let's not forget exhaustion: It's important to note that chronic sleep deprivation, only too common in new moms, can exacerbate and even cause the "baby blues."

How can I tell the difference between the "baby blues" and real depression?

One of the greatest challenges for women who have the "baby blues," is to be able to distinguish between the normal emotional fallout from having a baby and real, clinical depression. It's not an easy task because the symptoms definitely overlap. But here are a few key differences:

- **The timetable:** The "baby blues" usually occur right after birth and will resolve in a matter of a few days to a few weeks. A clinical depression can develop anytime after the baby is born and the symptoms tend to be longer lasting.
- **Severity of symptoms:** Going through the "baby blues" can be pretty rough, but most women who experience this emotional upheaval can go about their day without severe disruption. Women who are clinically depressed most often have more intense symptoms that get in the way of their daily functioning.
- **Risk factors:** There are no real risk factors for getting the "baby blues"; they can happen to any new mom,

especially because fluctuating hormones and stress are universal experiences right after the baby is born. For depression, on the other hand, there are some risk factors worth mentioning, though depression, too, can happen to anyone. Among the risk factors that make certain women more vulnerable are a personal or family history of depression. (See the next section on postpartum depression for more details.)

- **Treatment:** The "baby blues" usually go away on their own without requiring treatment. Postpartum depression, on the other hand, often requires treatment with medication and therapy before it resolves.

Any tips for making the "baby blues" easier to deal with?

Yes. Despite the fact that the "baby blues" will almost always disappear by themselves, there are a few things you can do to make life easier during this time period.

- Get as much sleep as possible. Sleep deprivation can magnify your feelings twofold. Try to nap with the baby if at all possible. If you can't sleep at nap time, take the time to relax, read a magazine or watch a good movie—anything that can give your mind a much-needed escape.
- Enlist the help of family and friends. If someone offers to babysit, take them up on it! Use the time away from the baby to take a walk, call an old friend, meditate, or go to a yoga class. Many women complain that they feel

so overwhelmed in the beginning that they forget about themselves completely. Don't let that happen to you.

- Remind yourself that these feelings are temporary. Knowing that there's a light at the end of the tunnel can really help. For most women, the "baby blues" will pass rather quickly, especially once the hormones level out.
- Network. Talk to other moms who have been there. Knowing that you're not the only one who cries, laughs, weeps, and cries again in a matter of seconds will make you feel a lot better. Many women who have experienced emotional turmoil following the birth of their babies will happily share their experiences with you. Just hearing that other women have made it through unscathed can help ease your anxiety.

POSTPARTUM DEPRESSION

Most women think it won't happen to them, but postpartum depression can strike anyone. It can affect women with a history of depression and women without one. And it doesn't discriminate. It affects women of all ages, races, ethnicities, and socioeconomic backgrounds. The only common thread is the birth of a baby, and even if a woman wasn't depressed with her first child, she can still become depressed after the birth of her second or third.

The cause of postpartum depression isn't fully understood, but hormones definitely seem to play a role. During pregnancy, estrogen and progesterone levels increase. Right after delivery, the level of these two female hormones drops rapidly. Scientists speculate that the swift change in hormone levels can trigger depression.

On the whole, women are more susceptible to depression than men, even when they're not pregnant or postpartum. Depressive disorders affect roughly ten percent of the population in the United States, according to statistics from the Society for Women's Health Research, in Washington, DC. What's more: Women are two to three times more likely than men to suffer from depression over the course of a lifetime.

While postpartum depression is not as common as the baby blues, studies indicate that roughly ten to twenty percent of women are affected. The numbers may actually be much higher, because unfortunately, postpartum depression so often goes undiagnosed.

Living with postpartum depression can be extremely debilitating. Some women have no energy and can't get out of bed; other women feel hopeless and start to withdraw from everyone around them; still others feel overwhelmed by having to care for a newborn, and unsure whether they love the baby enough. Women I've spoken with have described feelings of shame about their emotions: "How can I feel this way, when I have a healthy baby and a loving husband and everything I could possibly want?" Women who have gone through fertility treatments to get pregnant may have an added burden of guilt: "After everything I went through to get pregnant, I don't feel entitled to be sad now that I finally have a baby."

The tricky thing about postpartum depression is that it doesn't look the same in everyone. Feelings of stress, anxiety, and incompetence may also be signs of postpartum depression. One woman told me, "I felt like I was spinning out of control and unable to do anything right." Because fear and anxiety aren't typically thought of as "depressive" feelings, many women fail to recognize them for what they are, and as a result, they'll often try to deal with their emotions on their own, without seeking the proper help.

And it's not just the anxiety-ridden women who fail to seek treatment. One study of depressed new mothers estimated that roughly ninety percent recognized that something was wrong, but only one-third characterized their symptoms as postpartum depression. What's worse: Less than twenty percent of the women in this study sought treatment.

Despite the fact that recent media attention has shed light on this ailment, many women continue to suffer in silence, or else to be misdiagnosed when they do seek help. Unfortunately, untreated postpartum depression can have serious consequences. A mother suffering from depression may not bond as easily with her child. She may experience a lack of energy and difficulty concentrating, two common symptoms of depression, and unfortunately, two attributes very necessary to meet the demands of a young infant. Feelings of incompetence may ensue, which can aggravate already existing feelings of depression and create a vicious cycle.

And Mom's not the only one at risk. According to data from the National Women's Health Information Center at the United States Department of Health and Human Services, postpartum depression can have detrimental effects on language development and activity levels in infants. Some studies suggest that infants of depressed new moms may have a higher rate of sleep and behavioral problems.

Other members of the family may be affected too. Studies show that postpartum depression can have a negative impact on the relationship between a mother and her spouse or partner. Sometimes, the partners of depressed women don't fully understand the scope of the problem. I've spoken to several husbands who've asked me, "Shouldn't her symptoms have passed already?" or "What is she *so* nervous about?" Others expressed frustration with their wives' symptoms: "Why can't she just snap out of it? She's bringing our whole family down." If the marital relationship or partnership is affected, the depression can persist or even get worse.

When there are other children in the family, they can suffer as well. Many well-established studies have consistently shown that maternal depression can impact the entire family. One study from researchers at Columbia University revealed that children of mothers with untreated depression have significantly higher rates of anxiety, and disruptive and depressive disorders, which can carry on into adulthood. When Mom was successfully treated for her depression, the risk of developing emotional or psychiatric conditions decreased in her children, according to the study.

There is also some evidence that depression can affect the body as well as the mind. Untreated depression is associated with increased levels of cortisol, or stress hormone, in breast milk. And while more studies are needed to fully understand the effect, if any, on the baby, it serves to illustrate the powerful effect our minds can have on our bodies. When Mom is treated, the cortisol levels appear to return to normal.

For all the reasons just described, suffering in silence shouldn't be an option for women. The more awareness there is about postpartum depression, the better off everyone will be. Recognizing the symptoms and acknowledging this very common condition is important for mothers, fathers, children, and health care professionals alike. If you know someone suffering from postpartum depression, urge her to get the help she needs and deserves.

THE DIFFERENT FACES OF POSTPARTUM DEPRESSION: DEPRESSION AND ANXIETY

Does this series of events, which I call scenario one, sound familiar? You and your husband couldn't wait to have children. Ever since your honeymoon, you'd fantasized about becoming parents. You both grew up in sizeable families and longed to have a large family yourselves.

When you pictured motherhood, images of cherubic children filled your thoughts: children playing soccer in the backyard, eating hotdogs at family barbecues, and assembling their first words on Scrabble night. But the reality of having a newborn caught you off guard. From the very beginning, things were much more difficult than you ever imagined.

Your labor was terrible. It dragged on for hours and the pain was never really under control. You had two failed epidurals and by the time you were fully dilated, the pain was so intense, you were convinced a successful epidural wouldn't have knocked it out. And you pushed for more than an hour. When you finally gave birth to your son, you were totally exhausted and had been stitched up, with a third-degree tear that extended all the way to your rear end.

And things got worse when you got home. The baby had colic and would cry for five hours in a row. He didn't sleep well either. You wanted to breastfeed, more than anything, but that went badly too. And when you tried giving him a bottle because he always seemed hungry, he wouldn't take it. You felt frustrated, helpless, and exhausted. When your husband would leave for work in the morning, you'd cry hysterically. You felt isolated, alone, and sad. How could motherhood have turned out like this?

As the weeks dragged on, you didn't feel any better. When the baby cried, you'd lock yourself in the bedroom, daydreaming of ways to escape your life. You felt like you could do nothing right, which made you sad and more frustrated.

You stopped showering in the morning. *What's the point?* you thought. At your six-week checkup, you had an emotional breakdown in your doctor's office. She recommended a therapist and informed you that you were suffering from postpartum depression.

What are the most common symptoms of postpartum depression?

The symptoms of postpartum depression can vary from person to person. Because so many women expect to feel some form of the "baby blues," the signs of a real depression are often overlooked or missed.

Here's a list of some of the more common symptoms of postpartum depression:

- apathy or loss of interest or pleasure in activities
- lethargy or lack of energy or motivation

- persistent feelings of sadness
- feeling worthless or hopeless
- feeling overwhelmed or anxious
- repeated bouts of crying
- changes in appetite
- changes in sleep patterns
- feeling angry, irritable, or restless
- withdrawal from family or friends
- thoughts of harming the baby
- thoughts of harming yourself

Typically, if a person suffers from one or more of these symptoms for more than two weeks, she may have postpartum depression—even if some of the symptoms don't really fit into the conventional notion of "depression."

Why do some women get postpartum depression but others don't?

At this point, no one knows for sure. Besides postpartum hormonal fluctuations, which may affect different women in different ways, researchers have been able to identify certain risk factors which may contribute to a woman's likelihood of becoming depressed during or after pregnancy. These include:

- a personal history of depression or mental health problems before the pregnancy
- a family history of depression or mental illness
- a previous depression with other pregnancies

- severe premenstrual syndrome (PMS) or premenstrual dysphoric disorder (PMDD), a condition characterized by serious emotional and physical symptoms related to the menstrual cycle
- having marital problems
- being a single mom
- having a limited support network
- complications during birth
- having a baby with physical or psychological problems

It's important to note that not all women who have one or more of these risk factors will become depressed. But these factors do make it more likely that a woman will become depressed in the time period surrounding the birth of her baby.

When most people think of "depression," they often think of sadness and crying spells . . . .

But consider this, scenario two.

After you gave birth, your mom agreed to help out for a few weeks until you were up on your feet again. Your labor was fairly normal for a first-time birth, but you had a pretty extensive episiotomy which left you writhing in pain every time you needed to go to the bathroom. You were thankful for the extra help.

Your mom planned on staying two weeks, but you talked her into two more. By the end of the four weeks, you felt much better—physically, that is. But the very thought of your mother leaving terrified you, because you had come to rely on her—more than you wanted to. As the day approached, your mood started to change. The early euphoria of becoming a mother slowly gave way to anxiety and fear. *How can I do this alone?* you thought.

You remember holding on to your mother's ankles as she left your home . . . or was that a dream? Either way, it was how you felt. And as that door closed, you slowly turned around and saw a tiny infant in a car seat. She was so small, but yet, the feelings she elicited in you were so large. You were scared, and as feelings of panic washed over your body, you started to cry.

The panicky feelings lasted for weeks. No longer did you have the help you had come to rely upon so heavily. The sleep deprivation was taking its toll too. The baby woke you every two to three hours and you became worried that you'd be unable to care for her on so little sleep. You felt sorry for your daughter that your mother had left. You became obsessed with her sleep habits and your own. You walked down the street estimating on the basis of how they looked how much sleep other people were getting.

When the baby finally started sleeping for longer stretches, you couldn't. You'd been breastfeeding for the last few months and your body was trained to listen for her cries. You'd hear her even when she wasn't crying. If the air conditioner squeaked or a dog barked, you'd jump to attention, your heart racing.

You started to fantasize ways to get your mom back. Things were much easier when she was at your apartment. You missed your old life—the one where you were being mothered rather than having to do the mothering. If only your episiotomy wouldn't heal so fast; maybe you could break your leg?

What's going on in this scenario?

As discussed earlier, worry and anxiety may characterize postpartum depression just as readily as sadness and crying spells. Notice also how pervasive the feelings of worthlessness are in the second scenario. This person even "feels sorry" for her newborn once her mother has left, because she doesn't believe herself to be a good enough mother. These emotions, too, are typical of a postpartum depression.

It sounds like this woman is suffering from anxiety, not depression.

There is quite a bit of overlap when it comes to the symptoms of depression and anxiety. Studies show that postpartum depression symptoms can overshadow, or coexist with, postpartum anxiety. That means that women can suffer from both at the same time. Studies also suggest that postpartum anxiety is probably more common than we realize. The take-home message is: The symptoms in both scenarios are real and shouldn't be taken lightly. Both women should speak to a health professional about their symptoms, and both women will likely need some kind of treatment.

What is known about postpartum anxiety?

One thing we know is that over the course of a lifetime, anxiety disorders in general are more common in women than in men. And because of the hormonal fluctuations experienced after a baby is born, anxiety may be particularly likely in the postpartum period, especially in women who have suffered from anxiety at other times.

There are a host of different forms that anxiety can take during the postpartum period. They range from mild anxiety to full-blown panic disorder. Some women even experience symptoms of obsessive-compulsive disorder (OCD) following the birth of their babies. These women may have repetitive thoughts, which could include fear of harm coming to the newborn or even thoughts of hurting themselves or their baby.

Here is a list of some of the more common symptoms of the anxiety disorders that may occur in the postpartum period:

- constant worry that you can't take adequate care of the baby
- anxiety that gets in the way of eating or sleeping
- feeling on edge or restless for an extended period of time
- recurrent or persistent thoughts of harming yourself or the baby
- repetitive behavior or rituals that are invoked to relieve anxiety or stress
- panic attacks, which are characterized by a rapid heart rate, sweating, difficulty swallowing, shortness of breath, dizziness, pins and needles in the hands or feet, and/or a feeling of choking or dying

Why is postpartum anxiety so hard to spot?

What makes postpartum anxiety difficult to diagnose is that the vast majority of new mothers feel a little anxious or overwhelmed, especially in the beginning. Having a new baby is a life-altering experience, so it's no wonder there's a lot of anxiety surrounding it. If a woman's symptoms are getting in the way of her daily life, however, and preventing her from enjoying her new role as a mom, she may have a problem. Unfortunately, the symptoms described above are often dismissed by both patients and doctors. That's why it is really important for women to recognize them as serious and to alert their health care providers if they are experiencing them.

It's also important to note that certain physical ailments can cause the same or similar symptoms. For example, problems with the thyroid, especially hyperthyroidism, can produce anxiety-like symptoms, as can low blood sugar or certain nutritional deficiencies which may be common in new moms on the go. Health care providers should have these conditions on the radar screen as well.

What are the treatment options for postpartum depression and anxiety?

The mainstay of treatment for postpartum depression is therapy and/or medication. Antidepressants, a class of drugs used to treat depression, are often prescribed for women diagnosed with postpartum depression. They work by increasing the amount of certain neurotransmitters, or brain chemicals, available to those parts of the brain responsible for mood. Neurotransmitters are vital to normal brain function, including frame of mind, disposition, cognitive processes, and sleep. Antidepressants are designed to relieve symptoms of depression by restoring the chemical balance of the brain.

There is a wide variety of different antidepressants available, and the drug classes are categorized based on the brain chemicals they target. For example:

- SSRIs (selective serotonin reuptake inhibitors)—Well-known examples of this class include Prozac, Celexa, Paxil, and Zoloft.
- SNRIs (serotonin and norepinephrine reuptake inhibitors)—Well-known examples of this class include Effexor and Cymbalta.
- NDRIs (norepinephrine and dopamine reuptake inhibitors)—A well-known example of this class is Wellbutrin.
- Tricyclics—Well-known examples of this class include Elavil and Aventyl.
- Combined reuptake inhibitors—Well-known examples in this class include Remeron and Desyrel.
- MAOIs (monoamine oxidase inhibitors)—This class is currently used much less often than the other classes.

Like other medications, antidepressants have side effects. Selective serotonin reuptake inhibitors tend to have fewer side effects than the other classes and are prescribed more frequently, on average. Common side effects caused by antidepressants include headaches, dry mouth, nausea, nervousness, sleep disruption, and sexual problems. Tricyclics can cause blurred vision and constipation, and can affect blood pressure and heart rate. MAOIs have more serious side effects including weakness, dizziness, and trembling, and tend to interact negatively, and sometimes lethally, with other medications or foods—which is why they are not prescribed as often anymore.

Because of the possibility of side effects, which can range from uncomfortable to dangerous, and the possibility of interactions with other drugs or over-the-counter medications, it is always vital to tell your doctor if you are taking antidepressants. It is also wise to ask the doctor who prescribes your antidepressants about potential food, alcohol, and other dietary interactions. And if you are breastfeeding, speak with your health care provider about the safety profile of your prescribed medication and its effect on the breast milk.

Certain medications are tolerated better in some people than in others. If you experience an unwanted side effect, alert your health care provider immediately. Many different options are available, including switching the dose and changing the drug or drug class.

The use of antidepressant medication is not usually a quick fix. It may take a few weeks for the levels to build up so that the full effect of the medication is felt by the patient. Therapy is often recommended in conjunction with medication, and studies have proven this combination to be most effective. It's important to note that some women can be treated successfully by therapy alone, without the use of medication. Treatment choices depend on the individual circumstances and underlying factors which may contribute to the depression.

There are many different types of therapy available to women suffering from depression including:

- **Cognitive-behavioral therapy,** designed to help the patient identify and change thought patterns and behavioral patterns that contribute to depression.

- **Interpersonal therapy,** which examines how depression can be linked to emotional issues and relationships in a person's life.
- **Psychodynamic therapy,** which examines events and relationships in childhood and earlier parts of the patient's life.
- **Group therapy,** which connects people who are confronting similar issues and crises. Women experiencing depression and/or anxiety in the postpartum time period often find great benefit from the support of other women who are facing the same kind of emotional challenges.

The length and duration of therapy and treatment depend upon the needs and responses of each individual. On average, women stay on the antidepressant medication for several months, and when they are ready to come off, the dose is slowly tapered. Therapy can continue after the cessation of medication, but again, it depends on the individual.

Finding a therapist can be a daunting task, especially for women who are suffering from depression or anxiety. If you think you may be experiencing postpartum depression, you may want to bring it up with your ob-gyn, who can probably refer you to a local therapist who specializes in postpartum issues. Alternatively, you could speak to your child's pediatrician for recommendations. If all else fails, ask around in your neighborhood, or look for local listings in newspapers or online, for support groups and/or therapists.

The treatment of depression and anxiety tends to overlap. Usually, the anxiety will dissipate as the symptoms of depression improve with therapy and/or medication, requiring no additional management. But for some women with acute anxiety, extra treatment may become necessary. Therapy sessions may focus on controlling anxiety-provoking thoughts and behavior. And doctors can prescribe medications which are specific to the relief of panic symptoms.

If special anxiety medication is necessary, a class of drugs known as benzodiazepines, which include Ativan, Valium, and Xanax, are often prescribed to relieve anxiety symptoms. Many doctors treating women with postpartum anxiety will recommend taking one pill on an as-needed basis. Women with obsessive or compulsive tendencies usually respond well to a class of antidepressants known as heterocyclics.

How safe is the use of antidepressants while you are breastfeeding?

There is no real consensus on this issue. Many doctors, nurses, and lactation specialists feel that it is safe, while others aren't sure. What is known is that the concentrations of antidepressant medications in breast milk seem to vary widely. The amount of drug that a newborn gets exposed to can depend on several factors, including the dose of the drug, the rate the drug breaks down in the body (maternal drug metabolism), and how often the woman feeds the baby. Hopefully in the future, we will have more clear-cut answers. But again, if you plan on taking antidepressants or antianxiety drugs while breastfeeding, consult your health care provider to discuss the risks and benefits of any particular drug.

POSTPARTUM PSYCHOSIS

After the baby was born, you knew right away that something was wrong. You were a little nervous before the birth, but nothing like what you were feeling afterward. The whole scene didn't seem real to you; it was as if you were watching a movie of someone else's life. The nurses tried to give you the baby to breastfeed, but you were in a state of panic. A lactation consultant came in to give you support and when you told her how you were feeling, she told you that it was your hormones and it would pass in a few days. . . .

But it didn't. At home, you could barely sleep. You were preoccupied with thoughts of dropping the baby. You felt like a terrible mother, which only increased your state of anxiety. You read an article about a toddler who fell out a window and you couldn't get the thought out of your mind. You kept imagining that the child was your baby and that somehow you had dropped him out the window. You became frantic and walked around your neighborhood for hours with the baby strapped safely in the stroller, to try to alleviate your anxiety. You knew that your thoughts weren't rational, but you were too scared to tell anyone about them. You didn't want people to think you were crazy or unfit to be a mother.

Things have continued to get worse. You've stopped eating. You feel empty inside. You turn down invitation after invitation from friends for coffee, walks, and lunch because you have no interest in seeing anyone. You were barely making it out of bed when you realized that you don't want to live anymore. You've started contemplating ways to take your own life.

What is going on?

You are suffering from postpartum psychosis, a rare and life-threatening disorder that can occur after a woman has a baby. Studies reveal that roughly one or two women out of a thousand may be affected by it. Symptoms can develop anytime within the first three months after delivery, but most often occur within the initial few weeks.

What are the symptoms of postpartum psychosis?

The symptoms tend to be severe and can include:

- delusions, or false beliefs (for example: the baby is bad)
- feelings of panic and/or anxiety
- obsessive thoughts of harming the baby
- sleep disturbances
- change in appetite or refusal to eat
- hallucinations, or hearing and/or seeing things that aren't really there (for example: hearing voices telling you to harm the baby)
- thoughts of suicide

Many women with postpartum psychosis report that the symptoms came on suddenly, without warning. Some felt depressed prior to the onset of psychosis, but many others describe feeling "fine" before experiencing any symptoms at all. Often (but not always), women with postpartum psychosis do realize that something is wrong with them.

Why does it happen?

No one knows for sure what causes postpartum psychosis, but it is very important to realize that, just like depression, this is a real, clinical illness that can't be wished away. Some experts believe that the birth of the baby and the ensuing hormonal fluctuations can trigger an abnormal state in the brain. There is also some evidence that postpartum psychosis is linked to bipolar disorder, as the women often experience rapidly shifting mood swings, erratic behavior, and manic episodes.

Is anyone at risk for this or only women who have mental illness?

That's a good question. Studies show that women with a personal history of psychosis, bipolar disorder, or schizophrenia do seem to have a higher risk of postpartum psychosis. But it can also turn up in women who progress from postpartum depression into postpartum psychosis, and in women without any history at all of depression or other psychiatric issues.

It's important to note that women who have had one episode of postpartum psychosis are more likely than those who have never experienced postpartum psychosis to experience it again with later pregnancies.

I read a story about a woman with postpartum psychosis who killed her child. Her husband claims he had no idea she was ill. Is it possible he

could have missed the signs? They seem pretty obvious.

Actually, it is possible. Spotting the signs can sometimes be more difficult than you'd imagine because the symptoms tend to come and go, especially the hallucinations. Many women with postpartum psychosis try to hide their symptoms from others, either out of fear or embarrassment. And remember, new moms often spend so much time alone with the baby by themselves that family members may not realize something is wrong.

Here is a list of **red flags** for concerned spouses, friends, and relatives. Red flags offer clues or tips to an outsider that a loved one may be suffering from postpartum psychosis:

- Mom seems prone to rapidly shifting moods.
- Mom displays disorganized or erratic behavior.
- Mom seems intensely concerned about the baby's health and safety, or else displays apathy or no concern at all.
- Mom voices exaggerated concern that she is doing a bad job.
- Mom expresses delusional beliefs about the baby.
- Mom engages in any kind of talk about suicide or infanticide (harming or killing the baby).

If you or someone you know is experiencing one or more of these red flags, it may be a medical emergency. Do not delay getting help. Sometimes, women with postpartum psychosis understand that they have a problem and are in need of assistance. Other times, it's necessary for concerned friends or relatives to guide them into the hands of qualified mental health professionals.

Keep in mind that not all doctors are familiar with the signs and symptoms of postpartum psychosis. As a result, some women are misdiagnosed and not treated properly. Health professionals and loved ones should realize that delusions, hallucinations, and erratic, inconsistent behavior are red flags that may signal imminent danger. If for some reason or other, the doctor doesn't recognize the seriousness of the issue, it's time to find another health care professional who does.

What is the treatment for postpartum psychosis?

The good news is that postpartum psychosis is treatable. A full screening and evaluation by a mental health care professional are necessary to arrive at a diagnosis and determine the proper course of treatment. If a woman poses a potential threat to the baby and/or herself, hospitalization may be required.

Postpartum psychosis can be treated with a variety of medications including: antipsychotic drugs, antidepressants and/or antianxiety drugs. Women with postpartum psychosis should also work with a therapist in a one-on-one or group setting. Many women are able to fully recover with proper care and treatment. The duration of treatment varies from person to person, but follow-up and monitoring by a health professional usually continue long after the symptoms resolve.

SLEEP CYCLE PROBLEMS

The last four months have been a nightmare for you. You're getting barely any sleep and are completely exhausted. Wasn't it all supposed to get better after the baby came? During your first trimester of pregnancy your sleep was disrupted by your need to pee every five minutes. Your sleep improved slightly during the second trimester, but in the third trimester, you couldn't get comfortable in bed, especially at the end when you were "enormous." You loved sleeping on your stomach, but that was clearly not an option. And of course the first few months after the baby arrived were sleep hell.

But even now that the baby is on a more regular sleep schedule, the situation hasn't really improved. Granted, she's still waking up two times a night, but even if your husband does the middle-of-the-night feedings, you still can't sleep. And when you do occasionally manage to fall asleep as soon as your head hits the pillow, if the baby wakes you, it takes almost two hours to get back to sleep—at which point, it's already time to get up again. It's a vicious cycle and is wreaking havoc on your physical and mental well-being.

Why aren't you sleeping?

If you're asking this question, it might reassure you to know that you are not alone. Sleep problems are a lifetime struggle for many women and they tend to peak at certain times of life. Studies reveal that women report sleeping problems most often during periods of hormonal fluctuation: at certain points on the menstrual cycle, and during pregnancy and menopause.

Almost eight in ten women experience more serious sleep disturbances during pregnancy than at other times during their lives. Hormonal changes, heartburn, an expanding belly, and difficulty breathing and getting comfortable all play a role in sleep disorders related to pregnancy.

But the problems often don't end there. Many women are surprised to learn that after they have the baby, it doesn't necessarily mean their bodies will automatically go back to their normal sleep patterns. Hormone levels continue to fluctuate after delivery, and as a result, sleeping problems may persist for some women.

Are sleeping problems more common in women than in men?

More than forty million women and men suffer from sleep disorders in the United States, but studies show that, in general, women are almost twice as likely as men to experience insomnia. A recent survey by the National Sleep Foundation found that roughly fifty percent of women had difficulty sleeping prior to and during menstruation. On average, women report disrupted sleep for two to three days each cycle. These sleep changes can be linked to the rise and fall of hormone levels in the body. Add postpartum hormonal fluctuations and a crying newborn to the picture, and the problem goes from bad to much worse.

Insomnia is the most common sleep problem in this country. It includes all kinds of sleep challenges—the inability to fall asleep, frequent awakenings during the night, or waking up too early and not being able to go back to sleep. Many of the women who complain of sleep difficulties during the postpartum time period suffer from this last problem—the inability to get back to sleep once they are woken up. Whether it has to do with hormone levels, a heightened anxiety level, the feeling that you need to listen for the baby, or a combination of any or all of the above depends on the individual. It's also important to note that women who suffer from postpartum depression or anxiety may experience sleeping issues as a result.

I've always had problems falling asleep before my period starts. Is there a connection?

Probably. Women who experience sleeping problems during their menstrual cycle may be more likely to experience sleep difficulties during and after their pregnancies. But more research is needed to fully understand the relationship between hormones and sleep.

All new moms are sleep-deprived; how would I know if I really have insomnia?

While it's true that all new moms struggle with getting a good night's sleep—it comes with the territory—that's not really what we're talking about here. If you regularly experience difficulty falling asleep or staying asleep and these difficulties occur regardless of your baby's sleep patterns, you may have a problem. Many experts agree that an official diagnosis of insomnia would be given to women who experienced difficulty sleeping on a consistent basis for at least four weeks.

Postpartum sleeping problems can get in the way of your daily functioning, impair your motor coordination and thought processes, and add stress and anxiety to the long list of new mom concerns. So don't ignore these problems.

What can I do about insomnia?

The good news is that there's a lot you can do about it. While prescription drugs may sometimes be necessary if the problem goes on for too long, there are many other behavioral and lifestyle changes that should be tried before resorting to medication.

Here are some tips that may help you repair your sleep cycle:

- Avoid the late-in-the-day caffeine fix. Cut back on caffeinated beverages at least five to six hours before you plan on hitting the sack. Consuming caffeinated coffee, tea, or soft drinks late in the day can really do a number on your ability to fall asleep at night.
- If you are experiencing serious bouts of disrupted sleep, try to make up for the lost sleep with naps. Women who are waking every three hours to breastfeed or soothe the baby can get caught in a bad cycle that becomes a pattern they feel they can't escape. If you're not getting enough long stretches of sleep to sustain you during the day, carve out some nap time to catch up so as to minimize the toll exacted by sleep deprivation.
- Keep to a regular schedule. Our bodies crave routine, so try to go to sleep at the same time every night.

- Avoid doing last minute tasks and housekeeping chores before bedtime—they will only add aggravation to your day and get the adrenaline racing to your mind and your body.
- Create a calming nighttime routine. I used to drink a cup of chamomile tea and watch a *Sex and the City* rerun before going to bed. It was my little half-hour ritual, short but relaxing enough to help me drift off to sleep (most of the time!).
- Avoid watching the clock. How many times have you looked at the clock every five minutes, stressing because you can't fall asleep? This is the worst thing you can do. The anxiety over not falling asleep only makes it harder to fall asleep. If you aren't asleep in thirty to forty minutes, get up out of bed and do something else. Read a book, watch a sitcom (nothing violent or upsetting), take a warm bath, whatever it takes to change your frame of mind and help you relax. You can try again a little later.

If you find that lifestyle changes don't help and you are tossing and turning consistently for weeks on end, therapy and medication may be an option. Sleeping medication is usually prescribed for a short period of time and should always be monitored by a physician, especially if you are breastfeeding. If you are suffering from depression, antidepressant medication may be a better option, but again, speak to your physician.

Does breastfeeding have any effect on sleep?

There's a lack of scientific evidence on this topic, but I've spoken to enough women to conclude that breastfeeding probably does have an effect on the sleep cycle. When a woman breastfeeds, her body produces prolactin, a hormone that promotes the production of breast milk, but also interferes with the body's fertility hormones, in part by lowering the level of estrogen.

This low level of estrogen is the reason that ovulation tends to get suppressed during breastfeeding, but it may have other effects on the body as well. Just as the low levels of estrogen that occur in women during perimenopause and menopause are believed by many experts to be among the main causes of sleep problems at the time of these life changes, they may have the same effect on women who are breastfeeding. Still, it's important to mention that many women who breastfeed have little difficulty sleeping. Hopefully, researchers will look into this issue more in the future, so we can better understand how breastfeeding affects the sleep cycle.

Are sleeping drugs safe while breastfeeding?

To date, there are very few adequate or well-controlled studies of the effects of prescription sleep medications on breastfeeding women and their babies. There is some evidence, however, that the amount of medication excreted into the breast milk by many sleep drugs is low. Discuss the pros and cons of sleep medication use during breastfeeding with your physician to decide what course of action is right for you.

I have difficulty falling asleep because I get unpleasant feelings in my legs when I lie down; it almost feels like insects crawling in there. What gives?

It sounds like you have restless legs syndrome (RLS), a neurological condition characterized by numbness, tingling, or other uncomfortable sensations in the legs, and the uncontrollable impulse to move the legs when at rest in order to relieve the feelings. Lying down and relaxing tends to bring on the symptoms.

In many cases, the cause of RLS is not known, but we do know that women who are pregnant or have just had a baby and who also suffer from iron-deficiency anemia, are prone to having it. (See section on anemia, p. 33.) The symptoms of RLS are usually alleviated after the anemia is corrected by iron supplements. You should consult your doctor if you think you suffer from RLS.

I'm so tired I can't see straight, but my husband seems to feel that his long hours at the office are just as exhausting as mine at home. How can I get him to give me an occasional break from the baby?

One thing my husband and I fought about for a while after the birth of our first child was how tired we were. It was like some contest from hell: Who had bigger bags under their eyes and who had slept for the least amount of hours? No one wins this contest and we have now come to realize that we are both pretty tired. If you need to catch up on sleep, try alternating naps on the weekend, so you both have a chance to recuperate!

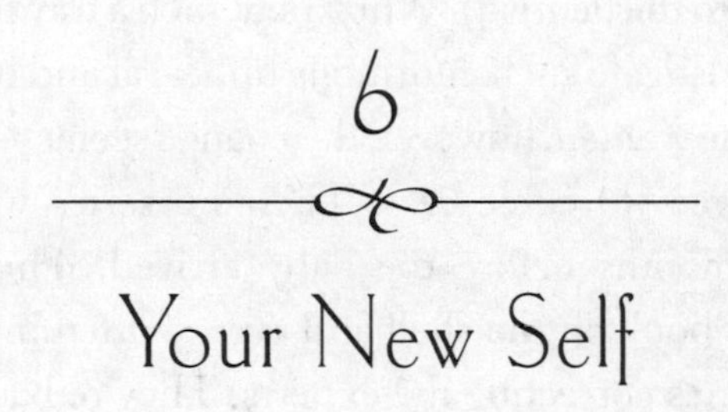

6

Your New Self

Probably more than just about anything else, adjusting to the "new you" can be the most daunting task you'll have to face after having a baby. As the craziness of the first few weeks passes and you finally have a chance to catch your breath, you may come to realize that your world has been turned upside down.

Everything has changed: your family size, your bra, dress, and shoe sizes, your schedule, your private time with your husband/partner, your private time with yourself, and most of all your sense of your priorities. After I had my first child, I was always struck by how little I had appreciated the ability to come and go as I pleased without really thinking about it: linger over dinner, catch a late movie, read magazines or books far into the night. These days are over once a child enters your life. Now, reading an article in the dentist's office prior to having a cavity filled seems like a treat (and I hate going to the dentist!). Who knew such a tiny human being could instigate such enormous upheaval and change?

For some women, however, the change seems—to an outside observer—to come easy. Their nurseries were decorated six months before the baby arrived. They've read every baby book on the shelf and even written into parenting magazines correcting the experts. They're back to their pre-pregnancy size and glowing with health two months after delivering. But don't be fooled. Every new mom goes through some sort of emotional mayhem; it's just that some of us are better at hiding it than others.

I remember when I first had my daughter I would take long walks on the promenade in Brooklyn, New York, and notice all of the other mothers strolling their infants. There was one woman in particular who seemed so put together. She had always taken a shower, had time to get an iced coffee, and from a distance, it even looked like she had had a pedicure (but I might have been hallucinating from lack of sleep!).

Anyway, she looked different from the rest of us new moms, most of whom could have been mistaken for the extras in *Night of the Living Dead.* I wanted to be like her, I thought. Until one day, I saw her on her cell phone crying hysterically to her husband, telling him that she felt lonely, isolated, and desperate to go back to work. She was still well-dressed and showered, but she was falling apart just like the rest of us. I cornered her the next time I saw her and struck up a conversation. Later, after we had become good friends, we talked about the emotional turmoil we had both felt in the wake of the life-altering changes that new motherhood brings with it.

After having many such conversations with other new mothers I realized that my friend and I weren't the only women having an identity crisis. There were others out there, many others, and none of us were as crazy as we thought we were. I started to recognize the power and security I got from surrounding myself with women in the same boat, so when my daughter was almost three months old, I formed a support group and hired a child psychologist to run it. Our membership filled up fast. Clearly, other women had similar needs.

There, amidst eight other exhausted, overwhelmed, and anxious women, I started to feel human again. Thank heavens for that one hour I could devote to myself each week; it truly kept me going. We discussed everything from breastfeeding and sex to constipation and sexism in the workplace. There was never a dull moment and never any silence, as the conversation often went well over our allotted hour.

Whether it's your relationship with your husband that takes a hit or the decision to go back to work that puts you over the edge, there's always going to be something that makes you feel that you're in over your head. It isn't easy juggling all of these new responsibilities in a world that offers so few accommodations to working moms, stay-at-home moms—or moms in general. One thing is for sure, many women have grappled with the issues you are facing. You are not alone as you walk the "new mom path"; it's a well-worn track, and you'll be much happier if you connect with some of the others who are on it with you. And sometimes your friends without children can be an even greater resource, because they may have more time for you than your friends with children.

LONELINESS

Many women feel a sense of isolation or loneliness after their baby is born. In today's world, women and men often live far away from other family members who could help out with childcare. As a result, the bulk of the responsibility falls on the shoulders of the primary caretaker, who is usually the mother.

Here are some typical expressions of loneliness from women I've spoken with:

> *We moved right after my first child was born to a town where I knew nobody. My parents live on the other side of the country and I hadn't had time to make any friends. My husband goes off to work each day and I stay home with our baby. It's been three months now, and I've started to feel really lonely. I love being a mom, but it's hard to be so disconnected from the rest of the world.*

• • •

> *I used to walk around in a daze from sleep deprivation and the shock of being a new mom. I remember looking into coffee shops longingly, watching working women chat with their girlfriends. I felt so alone, as though I was the only woman in the world without anyone to talk to all day long.*

A common time to experience feelings of isolation and loneliness is around three to six months. That's when the novelty of new motherhood has worn off and the reality that life has changed irrevocably starts to set in. And that's when many women need the reassurance of knowing that they are not alone in dealing with the stresses of being new mothers.

I've spoken to women who thought they were the only ones not having sex with their husbands; women who thought something was wrong with them because they didn't feel bonded to the baby; women who wondered if anyone else felt anxious about being alone with the baby. What they didn't realize was that there were hordes of other women out there going through exactly the same emotions at exactly the same time. Women need other women, especially after they've had a baby. They need to share experiences, laugh together, cry together, listen to each other, vent, and be validated. Here's another example:

> *I had the same routine every morning. I'd walk to the corner and pick up a bagel and iced coffee and go to the park. I hadn't realized that just two blocks away, Lisa was doing the same thing with her baby who was only two months younger than mine. When we finally connected, we'd go for coffee together and linger in the park for hours talking about our new lives!*

Networking with Other New Moms

The value of new mothers' support groups cannot be underestimated. They provide an opportunity to link up and feel connected with other women going through the same experiences. I've heard from countless women who have relieved their sense of loneliness and isolation in support groups, even when they met for only an hour or so once a week or every other week.

Check with your obstetrician for groups in your area or inquire at the pediatrician's office. If you can't find one, start one of your own. I did, and it was an incredible experience that brought new friends, lots of reassurance, and a wealth of practical information for dealing with all the issues I was facing. You can advertise in the local paper or put up flyers in local markets. Chances are you'll get a big response, because moms need each other, and the chance to connect can make all the difference in the world!

Staying Connected to Friends Without Babies

Some women feel a sense of detachment from their friends who don't have children. Before the birth, they were able to connect on so many levels, but after the birth, they wonder what they ever had in common:

> *We don't have anything to talk about. She rolls her eyes when I bring up the baby and the stuff she talks about seems so trivial to me. I can't believe we were ever friends!*

. . .

> *I used to meet my girlfriend every Tuesday for lunch before I had my baby. Afterward, the time didn't work for me anymore because it was during my daughter's nap. My girlfriend was not flexible, and as a result, I barely see her anymore.*

For many women, the demands that parenthood places on them can definitely have a negative effect on their friendships with women (and men) who don't have children. Sustaining these friendships takes time and energy, two things that get drained quickly when a baby is on the scene. But keeping up with good friends is important, and when you have a chance to catch your breath, you may regret not making the effort.

Keep in mind that someone who was a close friend before you had the baby may feel cast aside afterward. It's easy to get caught up in your new life and forget all about your old life and the people in it because motherhood can be all-encompassing. Don't assume that your friends without children no longer want to be a part of your life. Most likely they do and given the chance, will make time for you *and* the baby.

Here are a few tips for maintaining your friendships:

- Limit the "baby talk": While you may be enamored with every coo and gurgle, I assure you that many of your friends are not. They may be polite, but if your girlfriend doesn't have a baby, politeness can only go so far. Try to tailor the conversation to things you have in common. She'll thank you for it.
- Don't take the baby to social events unless you ask: One woman I spoke with was furious that she was asked to take her newborn home from a wedding rehearsal dinner. She hadn't asked the host. Err on the safe side and get a sitter. Or clear it with the party planner before making any plans.
- Set aside time to stay connected. Most every new mom will say she lacks time, but if you work at it, you can find ways to fit your friends into your schedule, no matter how busy it is. I always spoke to my friends on the phone while breastfeeding, and I tried to keep up with them over e-mail, as well. The little time you put in will

make a big difference. As the baby gets older, you'll find it's easier to stay connected. And you'll be glad you did!

- Put out feelers to see how open your friend is to spending time with you and your baby. Depending on the friend (and the baby, too), this may be easier than you think. A quick lunch at a baby-friendly restaurant, a walk in the park, a cup of tea at home while the baby is sleeping—all of these can allow the two of you to keep up your connection to each other, not to mention keeping you in touch with the outside world.

GOING BACK TO WORK—OR NOT

Your maternity leave is almost up and you're thrilled. Being alone with a baby every day is the hardest thing you've ever done and makes the worst day you had at the office seem like a picnic. Or, alternatively, you're heartsick about having to spend time away from your child every day but there is no choice; your family needs the income, end of story. If you decide to go back to work after the baby comes, chances are it is a decision you won't take lightly. Even if you're in the can't-wait-to-go-back-to-work camp, you still worry about how it will affect your baby. I've spoken to many women who grappled with this issue, stressing for weeks and months over it.

Obviously, there is no right answer; each woman needs to decide what's right for her and her family. But for most women, whether they are returning part-time or full-time, this decision is stressful, and sometimes heart-wrenching.

Take these experiences, for example:

Going back to work full-time was the most difficult part of post-pregnancy. I was not particularly psyched to be home all day and I knew I wanted to return to work. However, now that I've returned to work full-time I get calls at the office from my husband asking, "What is for dinner?" and "When are you coming home? The baby is hungry." On the one hand, this makes me feel extremely guilty, as though I am choosing to starve our child, but on the other hand, I feel really frustrated with my husband for not supporting my decision to work.

. . .

At five o'clock all I want is to be home with our daughter, but there are expectations at work that require me to travel sometimes, or to attend business dinners, or work late in order to hit deadlines. I am constantly trying to line up sitters and deal with the logistics of caring for our child when I am gone, pumping and storing breast milk, and making sure everything is taken care of. I get pulled in too many directions and feel like I am not being a good employee or a good mother. My husband and I have blowups when all this pressure and stress get to me.

. . .

I knew I would love our child, but I never thought that I would miss her as much as I do when I am at work. I frequently question if I am doing the "right" thing for her or for my marriage.

These sentiments are unfortunately all too common. Guilt, frustration, stress, and pressure often mount as women attempt one of the toughest balancing acts of their lives. And while there's really no way to eliminate these feelings, there are ways to cope with them.

Here's a bit of advice which will hopefully ease some of the stress:

Have a Talk with Your Husband

If you decide to go back to work, getting your husband on the same page is crucial. But it's not always that easy. Regardless of how "liberated" your husband may be or think he is, gender stereotypes that have been solidified through many generations are hard to overcome. I have spoken with many working women who feel that most of the burden of childcare, housework, and meal planning falls directly in their laps, even though they are putting in as many hours on the job as their husbands.

My husband has always been incredibly helpful, but I remember one time when I was taping a segment for a health show, and he called to ask me what to do because our son had just had a bowel movement while they were in a bookstore. I was in full makeup, rehearsing my lines, but had to stop in order to instruct him as to where to find a changing table (in the family bathroom, which was in the same spot it had been in since the store opened) and where to find the diaper bag (in the same place on the stroller where it had been for a year). I've told this story to a dozen women who have instantly identified with it and in several cases topped it with much worse stories of their own.

Your husband has to understand that you are a team, and despite the fact that you are (probably) the captain of the parenting ship, your "co-captain" needs to come aboard or else all of you may sink. Communication is the key. Try to avert blowups by planning ahead. You may want to sit down at the beginning of each month and divide up the tasks. Men tend to respond to visual props, so a list may be the way to go. Since you are both working, figure out what needs to get done and break it down together.

Here's a sample list:

- childcare
- bills
- garbage
- laundry
- housework (cleaning, gardening, shoveling, etc.)
- meals (preparing meals ahead of time can help, or cooking together, or buying healthy, ready-made meals)
- grocery shopping

Put initials next to each task. Doing this every month can keep you organized, and can also give you both the opportunity to switch tasks if it turns out that your current "choices" aren't working for one reason or another. Enlist the help of your partner and hopefully, he'll be willing and able!

Deal with Your Guilt

As if leaky breasts, lack of sleep, and stress weren't enough, you need to throw a large helping of guilt into the equation. Most new moms who go back to work after the baby is born experience the pangs of guilt. For some, they're little pangs; for others, the pangs could fill a football stadium. No matter whether you go back to work for financial reasons or personal reasons, full-time or part-time, guilt is likely to rear its ugly little head.

And it may not only be *internal* guilt. One woman told me that her mother-in-law scolded her for going back to work, telling her she would "permanently scar her child," even though the family needed the money from two incomes. Another woman told me that her husband continuously questioned her decision to return to work and implored her to reconsider.

While we may consider ourselves to be liberated women, many of us have more than our fair share of guilt and grief to deal with—from both external and internal forces. And although it's not possible to completely chuck the guilt out the window, there are ways to lessen it and cope with it (or at least try):

- **Arrange for good childcare:** Many moms worry that their children won't be well taken care of while they are at work. To alleviate this anxiety, do your research, which of course should include calling all references and questioning them in detail. You want to get a real sense of how your child will be cared for. Once you've found an appropriate caretaker and/or daycare facility, make sure that you and the caretaker are on the same page ahead of time by discussing your expectations and setting up a schedule. Finding someone who will accommodate your needs and provide a loving and safe environment for your child can make all the difference in how you feel about going off to work every day.
- **Don't try to be Wonder Woman:** This may be harder than it sounds. Many working women end up burning

the candle at both ends, often to the detriment of their own physical and mental well-being. Don't fall into this trap. After my daughter was born, a wise woman told me that I shouldn't expect to make straight A's in every aspect of my life. In other words, I could no longer be the model employee while striving to be mom of the year; something had to give. And while I resented this for a while, I came to realize that she was right, at least in my case. So do the best you can while you're at work, and then leave your job at the office when you go home so you can focus solely on your family.

- **Don't beat up on yourself:** Many women I've spoken with realized that they would be happier if they went back to work but felt guilty about making a "selfish" choice. If this is the case for you, realize that your child will be much better off with a happy, stimulated mom, rather than one who is restless, resentful, and bored. But if you do go back to work, remember to give yourself fully to the hours you spend at home. It's the quality of the time you spend with your child that will matter more than the quantity. So make those hours count.
- **Share the burden:** The logistics of childcare can be stressful. Enlist the help of your husband. Having two people to deal with scheduling and transportation issues can help alleviate the stress and burden.

Have a Plan If You Decide to Breastfeed at Work

Many women decide to continue breastfeeding after they go back to work. But this is another area that can potentially cause stress for new moms. Among other things, women sometimes wonder: Will the baby take the bottle? Where can I pump? Which pump is the best one? How can I store the milk? What if my milk supply dries up?

Wouldn't it be great if every workplace in the United States had on-site daycare? Unfortunately, we're a long way from making that a reality; so many working women are forced to either pump during the day or reduce feeding times to early morning and late at night and have a caretaker supplement with formula during working hours.

Here are some tips if you decide to pump at work:

- **Choose the right pump:** This is probably a good time to spend a little extra money because if you are going to pump at work, you'll need the right apparatus. Don't get intimidated because there are so many varieties to choose from. Just make sure you pick a high-quality, electric pump with a dual collecting system, so you can pump both breasts simultaneously and save time.
- **Practice makes perfect:** Don't try out your pump for the first time on your first day back to work! Get used to the pump for a few weeks at home before you return to work. This will help alleviate any problems that may arise.
- **Arrange for privacy:** This is an issue that you want to deal with before returning to work if you don't have an office of your own with a door that can be closed. Speak with your employer about arranging for a private room, preferably one with a lock so you don't need to stress about someone walking in on you. Alternatively, you could post an "occupied" sign outside an empty office. Of course, some workplaces

do have lactation rooms, but these are still relatively rare.

- **Find a place to store milk:** Stock up on storage bags and/or bottles. The American Academy of Family Physicians recommends storing breast milk in quantities of the size you can use at one feeding (2–4 ounce containers), because storing in too large a container may waste the milk. Breast milk should be placed in a refrigerator or cooler bag right away. It can also be frozen; check with your doctor or a lactation specialist for guidelines.
- **Don't forget the breast pads:** Conducting a meeting with two large, wet rings on your chest is not going to boost your employee rating. If you're nursing, wear pads and bring some extras along just in case.
- **Relax:** There is some evidence that stress can negatively impact your breast milk supply. Look through a magazine or listen to music while you pump.

If you choose not to pump at work, you can still breastfeed before you leave and when you get home. For some women, this works out really well. They are able to maintain enough milk for morning and evening feeds and not fill up and get uncomfortable during the day. Other women have a harder time. I spoke with several women whose milk supply became too depleted to keep up this schedule. As a result, they needed to supplement around the clock.

Having to give up breastfeeding when it's not by your own choice can be very upsetting. If your milk supply is waning and you still want to breastfeed, speak with a lactation specialist for tips. Together, you may be able to find a plan that works better for you and your child.

MARITAL STRAIN

It's no surprise that going from a two-person family unit to three (or four or five) causes disruption, especially when the original two are independent adults who are used to controlling their own schedules. Oftentimes, it's the birth of the first child that is the life-altering experience; by the time the second or third child is born, the lives of Mom and Dad have already been turned upside down and they've learned to adjust to the changes that come with parenthood. Other parents say that having two or more is not twice as challenging but ten times as challenging.

But whether you have one or ten children, it's always hard at first to figure out how to balance the needs of your child with the needs of your partner (not to mention yourself)—especially in the beginning, when the task of taking care of a baby seems so overwhelming. I've spoken with many couples who complain that their marital relationship takes a hit after the baby comes. Take these stories, for example:

> *My husband was wonderful at the beginning—very positive and supportive. Now that we are six months into being parents, I do think that the marital relationship needs more attention. We are on different sleep schedules which definitely affects intimacy.*

• • •

I really resent my husband lately. He gets home from work and is always too exhausted to pitch in. I know he's had a long day, but my day has been long too and by the time he gets home, I desperately need a break. I feel like I need to nag him just to get a little help. Most of the time, it's easier when he's not around.

. . .

My husband and I are teetering on the edge of separation. We made some mistakes as a couple, not protecting our relationship enough, not making and taking enough time for each other and ourselves, and not honoring those boundaries. As a result, our marital life suffered, and we found ourselves at very different places.

For many couples, adding a baby to the picture can produce stress. Recent studies have revealed that there is a higher degree of marital distress among couples with young children today than in the past. According to one study, a substantial amount of tension is created if expectations regarding shared responsibilities aren't met. In other words, couples fight about the unequal distribution of work surrounding the baby. I've spoken with many women who feel that their husbands' lives have basically remained the same, while their own lives have been turned upside down. Some women report feeling resentful toward their husbands because they feel they are the only ones making sacrifices.

Other studies have suggested that it's not necessarily that the baby creates tension in the relationship, but rather that the new role of parents stirs up problems that already existed in the marriage. Issues that may once have been easy to overlook all of a sudden loom large once the baby arrives:

I always knew my husband wasn't the fastest man on earth, but after our daughter arrived, his slow pace drove me crazy. I mean, how long does it take to change a diaper? My poor daughter would freeze on the changing table before he fastened the tabs. My mother told me to be happy for the help, but truthfully, I'd rather do it myself in half the time.

. . .

My husband has an expense account at work, which he uses regularly to entertain clients. It never really bothered me before, but now I can't stand it. It makes me nuts thinking he is out having drinks or playing golf, while I am home dealing with the baby.

Marriage counselors will tell you that between twelve and eighteen months after the baby is born is typically when many couples seek therapy. Making it through that first year is a milestone—baby is usually sleeping through the night, Mom's body has healed, and a routine is established—but once Mom and Dad get past the sheer relief of having survived, they start to wonder: What happened to us?

It hasn't been an easy time period for anyone: Sleep deprivation, mood disturbances, work issues, added financial burden, and sharing new responsibilities can all add up. At a time when the individuals in a couple need each other the most, the stress may have pushed them further apart:

I feel like we are two ships that pass in the night. We're going in such opposite directions. I can't remember a time when we focused just on us. I feel like I don't know him anymore.

. . .

Over the last year, I've felt closer to my girlfriends than to my husband. They know what I'm going through. They understand me better than he does.

And it's not just the women who feel estranged in the marriage. Men often feel left out, marginalized, and detached from their wives. Some men feel jealous of the baby and the amount of time their wives spend on childcare. Others feel threatened by the fact that their wives know how to take care of the baby so much better than they do.

She doesn't need me in the same way anymore. It's like there's no room for me when she's with our son. Sometimes, I feel like a third wheel.

. . .

I didn't know where or how to fit in. I like to be helpful, but I couldn't be there as much as I wanted to. My wife completely took over, leaving little room for me. And when I try to help, she just corrects me.

All of these feelings are normal and part of the emotional landscape of becoming new parents. Of course, not every couple will experience marital strain. But most couples will need to redefine their relationship and reexamine the roles that they now play as their family expands.

While it would be impossible to dispense advice that applies universally to every couple, there are several themes that do seem to come up time and again when talking to new moms. Here are a few things to keep in mind as you begin your journey down the path of parenthood:

Make Time for Each Other

- This may sound obvious, but the single most important piece of advice I received after I had my first baby was to make time for my marriage. With all of the demands of becoming new parents, it's easy to let the marriage take a backseat. Don't fall into this trap. Schedule time for each other and focus on the relationship that made you parents in the first place.
- Push yourself out the door (literally). Many new moms are reluctant to go out and leave the baby, even for a few hours. My advice: Do it! Find a relative or babysitter whom you trust and spend the evening with your partner. And make sure you leave the house. You may go kicking and screaming the first time, but the quality time you spend with your husband is worth it, even if it's just for a cup of coffee around the corner.
- Stay connected. I remember inundating my husband with information about my day the second he came home in the evening. By the time I was finished talking, we'd move on to other things without ever discussing his day. He later confided in me that he didn't think I was interested. I hadn't realized that in my excitement to share my day, I had neglected to ask about his. Other women I've spoken with have heard similar sentiments from their husbands. Make an effort to exchange stories on a daily basis so you can stay in touch with each other. You'll feel more connected, and if you're the one who's home every day while your husband is out in the world, you'll remember that there's life outside the new baby.

Every Captain Needs a Co-captain

- Many husbands feel marginalized, useless, or left out. Include him as much as possible when caring for the baby, even if you think he doesn't have a clue. Gently give him one.
- Bite your tongue. My husband used to jiggle my daughter on his lap every time she was fussy. She would be bouncing up and down on his knee like a bucking bronco, barely able to hold her head up. She looked carsick to me, but it did work occasionally. Your husband is part of the team, so let him help, even if you don't think he's as proficient as you are at certain things. Walk out of the room if you need to (as long as your child isn't in any danger). I know it's hard, but try.
- Be a team. Stay on the same page when it comes to parenting. This is just as important early on in your child's life as it will be later on. Studies have shown that consistent parenting styles result in less tension and conflict at home—both between spouses and with children.

Communicate

- Don't let tension build without opening up about it. If your spouse is doing something that bothers you or not doing something you wish he would, let him know. And encourage him to do the same. While it may be unpleasant to hear that you are a little too controlling—which is often what you'll hear—it's better to air gripes early so they don't snowball into monumental grievances later.

- One woman I spoke with felt like her husband didn't want to be intimate with her after the baby came. She lived with thoughts of rejection for months, but was afraid to bring the subject up with her husband. When she finally communicated with him, she learned that he didn't want to burden her with his sexual desires; he felt she was too exhausted for him to even suggest being intimate. After they spoke, they understood each other better, felt closer, and were able to meet each other's needs.
- Discuss expectations. Having a baby can create issues or bring concerns to the surface that you didn't realize were there before. Make sure you talk about what you expect when it comes to household chores, finances, sleep schedules, in-laws, sex, and parenting styles before problems arise. Knowing each other's expectations can ease tensions and pave the way to harmony.

7

Losing Your Extra Self

I was recently at a birthday party, when a woman approached my girlfriend, who had just had a baby, and innocently asked, "When are you due?" The look on my friend's face said it all. Although she claimed *not* to be upset, you could tell she was dying inside. After listing ten excuses for why she hasn't lost the weight yet—only three weeks after delivery—she looked at me desperately and asked, "Why haven't I been able to get back to my old weight?"

Women are so hard on themselves. After the baby comes, between feedings and catnaps, women tend to turn their attention to microanalyzing the physical changes pregnancy has wreaked upon their bodies. For many women, these changes can spark self-doubt, self-criticism, and feelings of hopelessness.

In the postpartum period, women feel they can no longer "justify" the extra pounds. After all, there's no baby in there anymore. Their once taut, expanding tummy is still large but sagging and probably covered by stretch marks, too. The sight can be downright depressing, and for some women, overwhelming. It's as if we have forgotten that we just carried a baby for nine months. Now that the baby is here, we want our bodies back, and we want them back now! Our partners may be adding to the pressure with either explicit criticism or thinly veiled displeasure.

But, as with my friend, no matter what you do—run a marathon, eat only grapefruits and Wheat Thins for two months, or wish on a shooting star—the weight doesn't miraculously disappear. Besides, those pounds need to come off gradually and safely. Starving yourself and/or overexercising is definitely not the answer. You've just had a baby, and your body needs food, rest, and more than a little TLC.

So how can you lose the weight without sacrificing your health? That seems to be the magic question. Some diet plans will promise new moms a slimmer waistline in record time, but you should proceed with caution. Rapid weight loss isn't healthy for anyone, least of all for nursing moms. Many experts recommend waiting at least two months before starting a diet, to give your body a chance to recover and, if you're nursing, to establish a steady milk supply.

Another reason to take those pounds off gradually is that there is some evidence that rapid weight loss can be dangerous to the quality of the breast milk. According to the US Department of Health and Human Services Office on Women's Health, environmental toxins that are stored in the body's fat can get released into the breast milk if a woman loses weight too quickly, possibly making the milk less healthy for the baby. In addition, some studies suggest that rapid weight loss can decrease a mother's milk supply.

And it's not just the quality and quantity of the milk that takes a hit. Women who deprive themselves of food and cut calories may experience fatigue, dizziness, and weakened immune system more often than women who consume the proper number of calories. Some studies suggest that women who diet restrictively in the postpartum period are more vulnerable to a decrease in bone mineral density. Extreme dieting may also negatively impair their mood.

For all of these reasons, the goal for losing weight in the postpartum period should be a slow and steady weight loss. Women who want to lose weight during this period should focus on good nutrition rather than stringent calorie restriction. According to joint guidelines from the US Department of Health and Human Services and the Department of Agriculture (USDA) published every five years, the average breastfeeding woman who wants to lose weight should not consume fewer than 1800 calories per day, from a well-rounded, nutritious diet. This will allow her to shed pounds gradually and safely.

But remember, everyone is different. Your individual needs may vary based on your pre-pregnancy weight, nutritional requirements, exercise levels, and a host of other factors, including whether or not you are breastfeeding. So before you start any type of diet or exercise plan, you should consult your doctor.

HOW TO SAFELY LOSE THE WEIGHT

Unfortunately, there's no magic bullet when it comes to weight loss after pregnancy. But even though the weight is not going to disappear overnight, with a little common sense and willpower, those extra pounds will eventually melt away. You just have to be patient and try not to get frustrated (I know it's hard). And while I'm doling out the advice, let me urge you not to compare yourself to your unbelievably lucky friend who was back to her pre-pregnancy weight and size six weeks after delivering. For most women, that's an impossible dream, no matter how hard they work at it.

But here's something that will help you (while also helping your baby): breastfeeding. According to some very convincing data from the La Leche League International, breastfeeding mothers who participated in a study had "slimmer hips and weighed less" at one month postpartum compared to mothers who formula-fed their babies. However, don't despair if you're using formula, because regardless of whether you are breastfeeding or not, you can get back to your pre-pregnancy weight.

The following are a few helpful rules that you should keep in mind as you're trying to do so:

- **Adjust your expectations:** Some women are surprised and frustrated that the weight doesn't come off right away. Realize that it will take time.
- **Don't begin dieting right away:** Give your body a chance to recover and build up a steady milk supply. Many health experts recommend waiting at least two months after delivery before starting on a new diet.
- **Make wise food choices:** Most new moms are hard-pressed for time, but that doesn't mean you should grab a candy bar or other low-nutrition, high-caloric

foods on the go. Choose foods high in nutrients, such as fruits, vegetables, and low-fat dairy products. Blend a smoothie with some fresh or frozen fruit and low-fat yogurt rather than indulge in a high-fat frappuccino at your local coffee shop. Take the time to eat right and you'll be surprised to see the way little changes can make a big difference!

- **Be aware of your nutritional needs if you are breastfeeding:** For example, women who breastfeed may experience a loss in skeletal calcium. Post-pregnancy diets that limit dairy products in order to achieve weight loss may exacerbate this trend and cause a further decrease in bone mineral density, especially if you're cutting out calcium-rich foods altogether. That's why it's so important to make proper food choices.
- **Don't eat your stress away:** I can't tell you how many women complained to me that they overate after the baby was born as a way to soothe their nerves or mood swings. Don't fall into this trap. Get up and exercise instead. Take the baby out for a walk or go for a jog. The exercise will do you good and help steer you away from emotional eating.
- **Aim for gradual weight loss:** According to experts at the La Leche League, breastfeeding moms who want to lose weight can safely shed about one pound per week. Like the USDA, they recommend consuming 1800 calories per day.
- **Steer clear of weight-loss drugs and restrictive diet plans:** This isn't the time for crash dieting. Food deprivation and weight-loss drugs have side effects a new

mom cannot afford, including headaches, dizziness, a racing heart, and dehydration, to name just a few.

- **Stay hydrated:** It's easy to forget to drink liquids and become dehydrated when you are multitasking and taking care of a newborn. But it's not healthy! Make sure to drink eight to ten glasses of water a day, especially if you are breastfeeding, which can further deplete your water reserves.

THE DANGER OF FAD DIETS FOR NEW MOMS

If you're looking for a quick-fix diet plan, you won't need to look hard. They seem to be everywhere, filling the shelves of bookstores, promising immediate weight loss in three days or less.

And these diets seem quite appealing to the legions of new mothers concerned with the extra pounds, praying that they will just come off already. Why not try a fad diet? What do you have to lose? After all, easy weight loss sounds appealing. And being thin has its health benefits, doesn't it?

Although losing weight has a definite benefit for people who are chronically overweight or obese, rapid weight loss programs are not the way to go for anyone, least of all new mothers. Aside from the health problems that fad diets can cause any woman, postpartum mothers have unique health concerns that cannot be ignored, especially if they are breastfeeding. For example, many new moms may be anemic. This is often due to the blood loss that occurs during labor and the depleted stores of iron in the body from pregnancy. Restrictive diets could further exacerbate a tendency to anemia.

Many new moms also suffer from exhaustion and sleep deprivation. Depriving yourself of food from any of the major food groups, as so many fad diets call for you to do, could contribute to headaches, dizziness, low blood sugar, nervousness, and nausea.

Another health concern for postpartum women is osteoporosis, a condition characterized by a loss of bone mass or bone density, increasing a person's risk of bone fracture. Today in the United States, roughly ten million people have osteoporosis and eighty percent of these sufferers are women. Both pregnancy and breastfeeding place particular burdens on a woman's bones. During pregnancy, all the baby's nutritional needs, including calcium, are dependent on the mother. If the mother doesn't get enough calcium in her diet, the baby will extract what it needs from her bones.

Bone loss can occur during breastfeeding as well. Women who breastfeed can actually lose a small percentage of their bone mass, which is usually recovered after breastfeeding ends. But if new mothers put themselves on diets low in dairy products, thus depriving themselves of calcium and vitamin D, they may be inadvertently putting themselves at risk of long-term damage to the health of their bones. And new mothers who choose to follow one of the ever-popular high-protein, low-carbohydrate diets may also be putting themselves at risk of bone loss and eventual osteoporosis, because there is evidence that high-protein diets promote the loss of calcium through the urine.

Take-home message: Steer clear of fad diets. Avoid

anything that promises rapid weight loss in record time. Even if you lose weight, you'll likely pack the pounds back on in record time once you stop the diet! Beware of any diet that prohibits certain food groups or that promotes one type of food only. Eating citrus fruits all day is not only unhealthy for your body, it will probably make you crave everything and anything else you aren't allowed to eat. So, do your research. Most of these miracle diets lack any real scientific evidence that they will work over the long term. And if you dig a little deeper, you may find that some of them have real health risks associated with them.

POSTPARTUM EXERCISE

Exercising after you've had the baby has many benefits. It can lift your mood, increase your energy, tone your muscles, and help you regain body strength. But you need to proceed with caution because having a baby is hard work, and your body needs a chance to recover.

Many new mothers wonder, how soon after I have my baby can I begin exercising? And what kind of exercise can I do? According to the American College of Obstetricians and Gynecologists, exercise can start as soon as a mother feels up to it. But this can vary widely from woman to woman based on the type of delivery she had or any complications which may have arisen. Some doctors permit an immediate resumption of light to moderate exercise for women with normal deliveries. Other doctors recommend waiting for the six-week checkup, at which point the doctor can make sure you are healing properly before you go back to working out. But women who have had difficult deliveries may not be able to resume normal activity or exercise regimens until well after the six-week mark. Check with your own doctor to see what's right for you.

In general, women who have noncomplicated, normal vaginal deliveries can safely resume their normal exercise routine by the six-week mark. After checking with a doctor, they should be able to engage in many different kinds of exercises including strength training, aerobics, swimming, and yoga. Women who have had more complicated deliveries may want to start with a simple walking program, then add some light strength training, and slowly increase the intensity of their workouts, avoiding anything that causes discomfort. For all women, pelvic floor exercises should be encouraged because studies show that they can reduce the risk of future urinary incontinence. (See Kegel Exercises. p. 175.)

Studies show that exercising at least thirty minutes a day can result in dramatic health benefits for your body, including weight loss. Some people believe that the only way to exercise properly is at the gym, but that isn't the case, and for new moms in a time crunch, it's not always possible. This type of thinking only makes it easier to forgo exercising altogether. I mean, who can squeeze working out into an already jam-packed day? But you *can* exercise effectively at home or around your neighborhood. You just need to make the time, set up an exercise plan that works for you, and go for it.

There are many different types of exercises to choose from. When getting back into shape, it's important to do a variety of exercises during your workout because each type can benefit your body in different ways.

- **Aerobic or cardio training:** involves any activity that uses large muscle groups and raises the resting heart rate above normal for at least fifteen consecutive minutes. The object of aerobic exercise is to get the body moving in order to promote health benefits for every part of the body including the heart, lungs, muscles, bones, and mind. Regular aerobic exercise also promotes weight loss. Examples of aerobic exercise include: walking, bicycling, jogging, dancing, cross-country skiing, and swimming.
- **Strength or resistance training:** involves activities specifically designed to build muscle and increase strength. This can be accomplished by lifting weights or using exercise equipment designed to build muscle. Strength training has many health benefits for the body including strengthening muscles, improving flexibility, burning calories and reducing body fat, improving posture and balance, and decreasing the risk for diabetes and high cholesterol. Strength training need not involve a trip to the gym. All you need is a set of dumbbells and you can do the exercises at home. Start at lower weights than what you're used to, and build up gradually. If you've never done strength training, it would be a good idea to have at least a few sessions with someone familiar with postpartum challenges.

As you begin to return to your old exercise routine—or embark on a new one—keep in mind some of the dramatic changes your body has undergone and how they may affect your workout:

- **Your uterus:** It takes at least six weeks for your uterus to shrink down to its pre-pregnancy size. During this period, the muscles around your uterus may be sore, especially if you pushed for a long time during delivery, so don't overdo it. Start off slowly with modified sit-ups, pelvic tilts, and stretching. If you experience any pain or discomfort, stop and rest a few days before trying to resume.
- **Vaginal bleeding:** Also known as lochia, it will be heaviest the first few days after delivery, but can persist for several weeks. While aerobic exercise is encouraged, a telltale sign that you are exercising too aggressively is an increase in vaginal bleeding or a change in color to bright pink or red. If you notice any of these changes, it's time to dial back the intensity of your workout. Try low-impact exercises such as walking, gentle yoga, or elliptical machines at the gym. If the bleeding persists, contact your health care provider.
- **Your joints and ligaments:** During pregnancy, some of your body's joints and ligaments have loosened to make room for the growing baby and to aid in delivery. These effects are still present after birth and can increase your risk of injury. So pay attention to the surface you are exercising on. Concrete and other hard surfaces can be tough on your joints and ligaments. Also, avoid high-impact and stop-and-go exercises such as step aerobics and kickboxing, especially during the first few months after delivery, until your joints and ligaments become more stable. Choose strength-training exercises because stronger muscles help you perform better with less chance of injury to tendons, ligaments,

and joints, which may be vulnerable and loose from your pregnancy.

Remember, overexercising too soon after delivery can cause some very unpleasant problems. I spoke with one woman who exercised too vigorously a few weeks after delivery, and she reported that her episiotomy stitches fell out prematurely. Several other women I spoke to experienced vaginal bleeding, partly from overexercising. Believe me, you don't want to be in these situations, so start off gradually. Also, if you weren't overly active before or during your pregnancy, don't jump into an aggressive cardio workout right away. Your body won't be up for it and you may do more damage than good.

Because every woman's delivery is different, there is no one-size-fits-all workout routine. Make sure to check with your doctor before resuming an exercise regimen after the baby is born, and discuss with the doctor exactly what you are intending to do to make sure the workout is appropriate for you. Once you are given the green light, here are some general tips for your postpartum exercise plans:

- Proceed slowly and cautiously and make sure to include warm-up and cooldown periods to get your body used to working out again.
- Start with fifteen to thirty minutes of low to moderate aerobic exercise which can include swimming, walking, or slow jogging, followed by muscle-toning exercises for your back, abdomen, and pelvis. (See Other Recommended Exercises, p. 175.)
- Try to exercise regularly. Most health providers recommend working out at least three times per week.

- Stay hydrated. Make sure you are drinking enough water (at least eight glasses of water per day). New moms tend to get dehydrated easily, partly because there are so many demands on their time that they forget to drink, and partly because of increased hydration demands if they are breastfeeding.
- Stop immediately if you experience any pain, vaginal bleeding, or ruptured stitches. Contact your health provider for follow-up.

Kegel Exercises

One of the most important postpartum exercises that you should do is Kegels. These exercises strengthen the pelvic floor muscles, which have been overstretched during delivery. Kegels are important to new mothers because they help regain muscle tone and can prevent urinary incontinence and pelvic prolapse.

Here's how you do them: Squeeze the muscles that you would use to stop the flow of urine. Hold for three to five seconds and then let go. Repeat ten to fifteen times. You should work up to a set of ten, at least three times a day. They should get easier the more you practice.

Other Recommended Exercises

Exercises that help strengthen your abdominal, pelvic, and back muscles are particularly important for new mothers because these are the muscle groups that have had to work so hard during pregnancy and delivery. The following will help you get them back in shape:

- **Pelvic tilt:** Stand with your legs shoulder-width apart, slightly bent. Put your hands on your hips and squeeze the muscles of your butt and abdomen, thrusting your pelvis forward. Hold the position for ten seconds and repeat ten to fifteen times.
- **Modified sit-ups:** Lie on the floor with your knees bent, your feet flat on the floor, and your hands crossed at the base of your skull. Raise your head and shoulders off the ground by tightening your belly muscles. Repeat fifteen to twenty times. Do not try to sit all the way up until your body is fully healed.
- **Buttocks lift:** Lie on your back with your knees bent. Lift your bottom off the floor and hold for five to ten seconds. Repeat ten to fifteen times.

As your body heals and you become more fit, you can make your workout more challenging by increasing the number of repetitions and adding new exercises. If you're not sure when to increase your exercise regimen, check with your health care provider for advice.

Special Concerns for Women Who Have Had C-sections

Few women who have C-sections will suffer from any long-term abdominal muscle weakness. But you should keep in mind that a C-section is major surgery and that the body needs time to heal. Also keep in mind that your abdominal muscles are used in almost every movement you make. If your muscles were cut or separated during surgery, you may face special challenges as you recover and before you start an exercise routine. During the first weeks following a C-section, remember to:

- **Rest:** Getting enough rest is imperative for all women who have just had a baby, but especially for women who delivered via C-section. Most physicians will recommend avoiding any physical activity at all during the first week.
- **Avoid heavy lifting:** It's important to avoid straining your abdominal muscles until they have fully healed, which can take up to six weeks. The muscles can get injured quite easily during this time, so avoid any heavy weight lifting at all costs.
- **Strengthen and lengthen:** At six weeks, providing the woman feels up to it, many experts recommend isometric exercises, a form of resistance training that involves contracting muscles without moving the joints. With isometric exercise you build strength by tightening groups of muscles in the body such as the quadriceps, the glutes (buttocks), the biceps, and the abdominals, holding for twenty to thirty seconds, and releasing.

When you're ready to resume a regular exercise routine, you should ask your doctor or health care professional for exercises that will help you regain muscle tone in your abdomen. Here a few examples:

- **Head lift:** Lie on your back with your knees bent and hands placed behind your head. Raise your head, bringing your chin to your chest. As your body heals, you can raise your head a little bit more each day, working toward bringing your head and shoulders off the floor, slightly curving your upper back. Repeat fifteen to twenty times. Eventually, you'll be able to do sit-ups, but make sure to check with your doctor first.

- **Abdominal exhalation:** Lie on your back with your knees bent, placing one hand on your abdomen. Slowly inhale (your hand should rise) and then forcefully exhale (your hand should fall), contracting the abdominal muscles.

Special Concerns for Women with Episiotomies or Lacerations

If you've had an episiotomy or any kind of laceration, you should not do anything to exacerbate the injury or delay the healing process. That means starting your exercise regimen slowly, and stopping right away at the first sign of any pain or discomfort. When you resume your exercise regimen, do fewer reps at a lower intensity if you are strength training, and do aerobics at a slower pace. Take whatever time is necessary before returning to a high-gear workout.

Special Concerns for Breastfeeding Women

While most medical research confirms that breastfeeding mothers can safely exercise, the physical state of the breasts shouldn't be ignored. Falls are a potential problem during exercise because enlarged breasts may throw off your center of gravity. So be careful not to change direction too quickly during exercise or do anything else that could throw you off balance. In addition, during the early days of breastfeeding, when women tend to suffer from pain and tenderness in the breasts, you may want to avoid any exercises that could exacerbate your discomfort. It's also a good idea to feed the baby before you exercise. Breasts that are empty won't cause as much discomfort as when they are heavy and full. And don't forget to buy a good nursing sports bra that gives you enough comfort and support!

Special Concerns for Women Who Are Anemic

New moms who suffer from anemia need to be especially cautious while exercising. As mentioned previously, the oxygen-carrying capacity of the body's cells is compromised by anemia and exercising too vigorously can cause dizziness, heart palpitations, shortness of breath, and fatigue. While exercising is not discouraged for women with anemia, be aware that your exercise tolerance may be affected by the condition. Take precautions, if necessary.

Special Concerns for Women with *Diastasis Recti*

Some women experience *diastasis recti*, a condition in which vertical pairs of abdominal muscles, which meet at the midline, begin to separate due to stretching or pressure on the abdominal wall. Though it is more likely to occur during the second or third trimester of pregnancy, as the uterus gradually expands, it can also happen during labor and delivery. It is usually painless and often manifests as a ridge extending down the midline of the belly. It can be diagnosed during a physical exam by the doctor. The condition is more often seen in women who have had multiple pregnancies because the muscles have been stretched multiple times.

The condition usually continues long after delivery and can cause lower back pain and poor posture. Special abdominal exercises can speed the healing process and encourage the sides of the muscles to come back together. Speak with your health care provider if you think you have *diastasis recti*. She will be able to recommend an exercise regimen that can help your body heal properly.

8

Defending Yourself from Your Child's Diseases

The first six months of my daughter's life, I never gave a thought to colds, stomach flus, or viruses. So when she seemed to be coming down with a cold for the first time, I was caught off guard. The next day, she had a fever and I took her to the pediatrician. "It's a virus," the doctor declared. "There's really nothing to do. Just treat her for the fever, and don't forget to prop up her head and use a humidifier to help relieve the congestion in her sinuses."

It sounded easy enough. But it took me two hours to pick out the right humidifier and another hour to prop up the mattress in the crib. After giving her Motrin for the fever, we were good to go—all in under four hours. But she was miserable, bleary-eyed, red-nosed, and exhausted from lack of sleep.

For several nights running, she woke up throughout the

night, and I stayed up with her to rock her back to sleep. We suffered through that first virus together. But finally, after a few days, she was starting to feel better, and I was so relieved.

Until—I caught it! My throat hurt and I was achy and congested. While taking such good care of my daughter, I had totally forgotten about myself. I didn't realize that all of the kisses and snuggles I'd been lavishing on her during our middle-of-the-night miseries had actually put me at risk for getting sick too. I just wanted her to feel better and hadn't paid much attention to washing my hands or sharing food with her. So, I had to pay the price. And she did too, because now we were both sick, and my husband, who was a medical resident at the time, couldn't really help out. As the primary caregiver, I became weak, tired to the point of exhaustion, and cranky.

My friend with older kids told me that when one of her kids is sick, everyone gets it. It's inevitable. *Yikes!* I thought, and wondered if it really is inevitable.

What I've learned is that it is *not* inevitable. As moms, we need to take care of ourselves for us and for everyone else. If we do, we have a good chance at staying well, which is important, because being a tired, sick, worn-out mom is an awful experience. Can you think of anything less pleasant than having the stomach flu, and repeatedly running to the bathroom to vomit while trying to rewind the fifth episode of Elmo for your sick child—who has just vomited all over the couch? You're miserable, and, worse still, you may not be able to mother your child as well as you would like.

Maybe you are like me. I used to believe in "super mommy immunity," a term I made up to describe the idea that somehow we were immune to our children's sicknesses. I thought that getting sneezed on, coughed on, wiped on, and open-mouth kissed would somehow magically pass through me—because it *had* to.

Reality check: We are not immune. Many of your child's illnesses can get you sick too, so take the proper precautions, because when your little ones are sick—and they will get sick, much more often than you were expecting, probably—they need some extra TLC, which is hard to dole out when you yourself have caught a cold, or pinkeye, or a case of the runs, or one of those projectile-vomiting stomach flus.

Children get sick so often because their immune systems aren't fully formed and because they spend so much of their time in groups. Think about it: They play on playgrounds, and go to daycare and playgroups, and everywhere they go they share toys with other children. Their cute little hands touch everything in sight and end up in their cute little mouths. It's not surprising that their infectious diseases spread like wildfire through the group.

The most common results of all this sharing and touching are upper respiratory infections—better known as colds—which are caused by a host of different viruses. On average, young children get six to eight colds a year, compared to adults, who get roughly two to four, according to statistics from the Mayo Foundation for Medical Education and Research. A child tends to suffer from cold symptoms longer than an adult. Remember, no matter what type of infectious disease your child has, the best way to prevent it from spreading to you is to wash your hands with soap and water (or an antibacterial soap or wipe) after every contact. Never share food or drinks, keep toys clean after your child has played with them by washing in warm, soapy water, and wipe up germs in the playroom, kitchen, and bathroom with disposable towels.

Besides colds, there are a number of common and contagious childhood illnesses that can land you in bed, at the doctor's office, or on your knees in front of a toilet bowl. Let's take a look at the ones that occur most frequently, each of which I've described in the following pages, along with tips that will help you cut your risk of catching one of these doozies from your child.

PINKEYE

You have just brought the new baby home when your three-year-old complains that her eye hurts. She's been rubbing it nonstop, but you haven't really had the chance to look at it.

The next morning she wakes up and there is gooey, yellow stuff on her eyelids. The white of her left eye is pretty red and she tells you that it itches. You wipe her eye with a warm washcloth and then run to the baby, who has just woken up from a nap and needs to be fed.

What is pinkeye?

Pinkeye, also known as conjunctivitis, is an irritation of the white part of the eye and lining of the eyelid. It's very common and can be caused by a host of different things, including bacteria, viruses, allergies, and irritants (dust, chlorine, smoke, etc.).

What are the symptoms?

Pinkeye causes redness in one or both eyes. People with pinkeye usually complain that their eyes are itchy and/or painful. Pus or discharge can make the eyelids stick together, especially in the morning when a person wakes up. If it's caused by bacteria, thick pus (yellow or green) is usually present. If a virus is to blame, the discharge tends to be clear in color and watery. Allergies or irritants will usually not produce a discharge.

Is it contagious?

Contagious is an understatement. Pinkeye, whether caused by a virus or bacteria, can be very easily transmitted to other household members, including you and the newborn. Moms most typically catch pinkeye from their children after they wipe the child's infected eye and subsequently touch their own eyes. Other kids in the house can catch it by playing with toys or using towels, washcloths, or utensils touched by a child who has pinkeye. Some parents may not realize how contagious it is: Just lying on the pillowcase of an infected person can transmit pinkeye, so it's important to take precautions.

How long does pinkeye typically last?

If pinkeye is caused by a virus, it typically lasts about a week to ten days, but symptoms tend to improve within the first five days. Once the symptoms disappear, a person with viral pinkeye is considered to be noncontagious. If it is caused by a bacteria, antibiotics generally cure most cases in about three to five days. After one full day of treatment with antibiotics, children with bacterial pinkeye are no longer considered to be contagious.

How can you prevent pinkeye from spreading through the household?

The first and foremost preventative measure is to wash hands. You should encourage your three-year-old to wash her hands throughout the day and to avoid rubbing the infected eye. The same goes for you. Wash your hands every time you have contact with your child, especially after you wipe the eye or apply compresses.

Here are some other tips for preventing the spread of the pinkeye infection:

- Don't let your child share wipes, towels, washcloths, or a crib or bed with anyone else. This can promote the spread of infection.
- Disinfect toys and other items commonly shared among household members.
- Disinfect television remote controls, phones, doorknobs, and other commonly touched items in the house.

These measures should help lower your chances of getting pinkeye. But watch for the symptoms in yourself and other family members and seek medical attention if you suspect you have it. You might need a prescription to clear the infection.

How is pinkeye treated?

Medicines are not usually prescribed for viral pinkeye, but the symptoms can be treated in order to make the person feel more comfortable. Use a clean washcloth, or warm or cold compresses (depending on which one the person prefers) to alleviate pain. Always use two separate cloths—one for each eye—to avoid spreading the infection from one eye to the other. Over-the-counter pain relievers such as acetaminophen and ibuprofen can also be used to make the eye(s) feel more comfortable.

Bacterial pinkeye is usually treated with antibiotic drops or ointments that need to be prescribed by a health care provider. Never use an old prescription to treat a new case of pinkeye without asking your doctor. The treatment is typically given several times a day for about a week.

THE CROUP

You're in a deep sleep when you hear something that sounds like a small dog barking. It's 3:05 A.M. and you're disoriented; you try to go back to sleep when you remember that you don't have a small dog. You sit up in bed. Maybe it's a dream? But, there it is again.

You walk down the hall into the baby's room. It's not a dream. The baby is awake, crying, and having difficulty breathing. You panic. You wake your husband, call the pediatrician, and breathe into a paper bag while waiting for the phone to be answered. The on-call doctor tells you to relax; the baby probably has the croup, which usually isn't serious.

She recommends filling the bathroom with steam and bringing the baby in to help her breathe more easily. You're told to make a follow-up appointment in the morning.

It works, the baby calms down, and everyone goes back to sleep. The scary cough goes away in a matter of days. The baby is left with a runny nose and a more normal sounding cough, and so, alas, are you.

What is the croup?

The croup is infamous among parents because the barking cough it produces can sound pretty scary. It involves inflammation and swelling of the upper airway and most commonly affects young children between the ages of three months to five years. Outbreaks of the croup often occur during the winter and early spring.

Viruses are the main cause of the croup, especially one called parainfluenza virus. Less frequently, allergies and some types of bacteria can cause the croup too. Even though it can be frightening for both parents and children, the vast majority of cases resolve on their own and can be treated at home.

Please note: You should seek medical attention if the symptoms do not disappear within thirty to forty-five minutes of treating with steam. Also, if your child starts drooling or has difficulty swallowing, trouble breathing (especially after you've calmed her), or has blue lips and fingernails, contact your doctor. A rare disease called epiglottitis, an inflammation of the cartilage that covers the windpipe, can mimic the symptoms of the croup. It is caused by the bacteria *Haemophilus influenzae,* but infants are routinely vaccinated against it so it's unlikely you will encounter this.

Can grown-ups get the croup?

Yes. If exposed to a child with the croup, most adults will get a cold. The same is true for older children exposed to the croup. Remember, the croup is usually caused by a virus, and viruses can be very contagious. Young children are particularly vulnerable to the croup because their airways are smaller and narrower than older children and adults. Don't be fooled: Just because you're not barking like a dog, doesn't mean you didn't catch something.

How would I know if I caught it?

If you have coldlike symptoms—including runny nose, congestion, cough, and a sore throat—within a few days of your child's bout of the croup, it is likely that you caught it. Parainfluenza and the other viruses responsible for the croup are often mild in adults but they can also cause more serious symptoms such as persistent coughs and pneumonia. So be careful and take precautions!

Are there ways to prevent it from spreading?

It's not so easy to take the trouble to wash your hands after being woken up at three o'clock in the morning. All you want to do is crawl back into bed. But you need to. Washing your hands is the most effective way to eliminate the spread of viruses that can cause the croup.

Here are a few other tips:

- Promptly discard dirty tissues or anything else used to wipe drooling mouths and runny noses. And don't forget to wash your hands! I can't tell you how many mothers I've spoken to who don't wash their hands after helping their children wipe or blow their nose!

- Don't kiss your child on the face while she has the croup. (When you want to dole out love, kiss the top of her head instead!)
- Wash toys with hot water and soap. This will lower the chances of other children in the house catching the croup.

STREP THROAT

Your son is miserable. He's not eating and has a fever. You noticed a red rash under his arms. Last night, he woke up and you noticed that he has bad breath.

The doctor told you to bring him in. On exam, he noticed that your son has swollen lymph nodes in his neck and white patches in the back of his throat. The doctor suspects strep throat and sends him for a rapid strep test. Sure enough, the test comes back positive fifteen minutes later. Your son is started on a course of antibiotics.

What is strep throat?

Strep throat is an infection caused by bacteria known as group A streptococci. People of any age can get strep throat, but it is most common among school-age children and teenagers. Symptoms include: a sore throat, fever, difficulty swallowing, swollen lymph nodes and occasionally loss of appetite, headache, and a rash. Children with strep throat often have a foul-smelling odor in their mouth.

What is the treatment for strep throat?

Most sore throats are caused by viruses and will resolve on their own in a matter of days, up to a week. But strep throat, which accounts for a smaller number of cases, is caused by a bacterium and requires a course of antibiotics to clear up the infection.

Strep bacteria seem to thrive in group settings like day care centers and schools—places where people are in close contact. It's important to treat strep throat promptly because if left untreated, it can cause complications in other parts of the body including the kidneys, joints, and heart.

How contagious is it?

Strep throat is quite contagious and can easily spread from family member to family member. Sometimes a person with strep has cold symptoms and when he/she coughs or sneezes, the bacteria can get transmitted. Strep can also spread when a healthy person handles objects, toys, utensils, etc., touched by an infected person.

Some moms are so busy caring for a sick child they fail to realize that they themselves have become sick. If you get it, you will probably feel ill within a few days to a week after being exposed to the bacteria.

Is my child still contagious during treatment?

Yes, but only for the first twenty-four to forty-eight hours. After that, most medical professionals would agree that a child is no longer contagious. But don't run out and share an ice-cream sundae! It's better to be safe than sorry!

Continue to take the necessary precautions to keep yourself and other family members healthy.

I thought the strep had disappeared, when my son developed a rash all over his body. Is it still the strep or could it be something else?

It sounds like scarlet fever, another type of group A strep disease which can follow a throat infection. Scarlet fever typically produces a "sandpaper rash," made up of small red dots that are rough in texture. In some cases, the face flushes and the tongue turns bright red. Scarlet fever can be treated with antibiotics. Sometimes people experience skin peeling on their fingers and toes after the infection resolves.

How can you prevent strep throat from spreading?

Make sure to wash your hands. And teach your children to do the same. If you have school-age kids, you could pack an antibacterial hand sanitizer or wipes for school and encourage them to use them before eating. Washing hands with soap or using an alcohol-based hand sanitizer have both proven effective in preventing the spread of bacteria including streptococcus.

Here are a few other tips that may help:

- Teach your child to cover his/her mouth and nose when coughing and sneezing.
- If you wipe your child's nose, discard tissues and thoroughly wash your hands.

- Make sure to wash all plates, sippy cups, bottles, forks, and spoons in the dishwasher and don't forget to wash your own hands after placing the items in the dishwasher.
- Disinfect all toys used by the infected child to avoid the spread to other children.

PARVOVIRUS ("FIFTH DISEASE")

You thought it was just a cold. Your daughter has a low-grade fever and a runny nose. And all she wants to do lately is lie on the couch and watch movies.

She seemed to be getting better, but today she woke up with a bright red cheek, which looks like a rash. You noticed some red splotches on her arms and trunk too. Now you're not sure what she has.

Is it more than a cold?

It sounds like your daughter has parvovirus, also known as "fifth disease." Despite its name, it is not a disease, it's a mild viral illness which typically produces a low-grade fever, a stuffy and/or runny nose, and a lack of energy.

A few days after the coldlike symptoms resolve, a rash can develop which often begins on one or both cheeks and spreads down the body to the trunk, arms, and legs. The facial rash often looks like the child has been slapped on the cheek (or cheeks). It may take a few weeks for the rash to completely fade away.

Can adults get it?

Yes. If an adult hasn't been previously infected by the virus, he/she can catch parvovirus from an infected person. Parvovirus is most contagious when a child has cold symptoms, before the rash breaks out. Most studies suggest that once the rash appears, the illness is no longer contagious.

In some adults, parvovirus can be asymptomatic (have no symptoms); in others, it can cause serious fatigue, joint swelling, joint or muscle pain, and a rash. Joints of the wrists, hands, and knees, on both sides of the body, are the ones most often affected. Joint involvement typically lasts a few weeks but can persist for several months. Some studies have shown that women are more susceptible than men to joint pain and swelling if infected by the virus.

Once you get parvovirus, are you immune?

Yes. Once you have had fifth disease, you cannot get it again. According to statistics from the Centers for Disease Control and Prevention, roughly fifty percent of adults have been infected with parvovirus and are therefore immune. Young children are more likely to get it from each other, because they haven't been exposed yet.

I've heard that fifth disease can be serious; is that true?

For most people, it isn't serious; the symptoms are often so mild, many people don't even realize they have anything. It is worth noting, however, that in some women the joint pain can be quite debilitating. I spoke to one woman who had difficulty moving her wrist but didn't know what was wrong. She was worked up for all sorts of autoimmune diseases including rheumatoid arthritis and lupus. Needless to say, after quite a scare, she was relieved to be diagnosed with parvovirus. So, if you suffer from joint pain or swelling after your child has parvovirus, this diagnosis should be on your radar screen.

What is the treatment for parvovirus?

Because parvovirus is caused by a virus, antibiotics are of no use. Depending on the symptoms, doctors may recommend pain relievers, fluids, activity restriction, and rest. If a person with an underlying chronic illness gets infected by parvovirus, additional treatment may be necessary.

What if you're pregnant and you get it?

Parvovirus is particularly dangerous for pregnant women, especially those in the first trimester of pregnancy. If exposed, the mom can pass on the virus to the fetus, and in a small number of cases, it can cause a miscarriage. Luckily, half of all pregnant women are immune to parvovirus and severe complications in those who are not immune are quite rare.

If you are pregnant and have been exposed to parvovirus, it would be wise to consult your health care professional. She may want to monitor your pregnancy or offer other treatment options.

It's important to note that parvovirus can also be

dangerous for people with hemolytic anemia (like sickle cell anemia). So if you fall into that category and have been exposed, you should speak with your doctor.

How can you stop the spread of parvovirus?

As with all other viruses, hand-washing is imperative. The simple act of washing your hands frequently can dramatically cut your chances of getting parvovirus. Remember, the illness is most contagious when your child has coldlike symptoms, so make sure to take the proper precaution in time.

IMPETIGO

Your child has a red sore under his nose and above his mouth. It looks a little like a pimple. It doesn't seem to bother him, but the next day, you notice some clear fluid leaking out of it. It starts to crust over, when you notice another red sore starting to form near his mouth. You're not sure what to make of it, so you call the doctor who tells you it sounds like impetigo.

What is impetigo?

Impetigo is a common skin infection that most frequently affects infants and young children. It is caused by bacteria that live on the skin, either staphylococcus or streptococcus. When the skin gets damaged by a cut or insect bite, for example, the bacteria can make their way through the skin and cause an infection.

It typically begins as a red sore, which [illegible] and break open, releasing a clear or clou[illegible] brown crust forms fairly quickly and then [illegible] Impetigo is most often seen on the face, arou[illegible] mouth.

Can adults get it?

They sure can. Impetigo is most often seen in young children, but adults can get it too. Contact with an infected person, or with something an infected person touched, can spread impetigo. So moms need to be careful, especially when caring for a child with open sores.

It's important to note that impetigo can easily spread to other areas of the body, if a child continuously scratches the sores.

Is it serious?

Not usually. Most cases of impetigo resolve without any serious complications. Sometimes, mild cases just need to be monitored and will go away on their own. But remember, you're dealing with bacteria which can spread to other areas of the body. So you'll want to take your child in to see the doctor who can best determine the proper course of action.

What is the treatment for impetigo?

Many cases of impetigo can be treated with an antibiotic ointment, which needs to be prescribed by a doctor. If the infection doesn't respond or it spreads to other areas of the body, an oral antibiotic may become necessary. Always finish he entire course of antibiotics, even if all of your symptoms have resolved. Stopping short can result in the infection coming back, sometimes with a vengeance!

How can you prevent impetigo from spreading among family members?

Encourage everyone in the house to wash their hands with soap and water and to dry their hands and face with their own towels. The person who has impetigo should not use a regular towel but should be given paper towels instead, especially while the infection is healing, and should dispose of the paper towels promptly in a place where no one else will come in contact with them. Avoid sharing pillows, blankets, toys, and other items until everyone is healthy. Remember to wash all laundry from the infected person separately and on the hottest cycle possible.

CHICKEN POX

Your son just got vaccinated for the chicken pox. A few days later, you noticed some red spots on his back. You ignored them because you've been spending a lot of time outside, and you thought the spots looked like bug bites. But a few days after that, the spots seemed to change. Now they were fluid-filled blisters; a few had opened and were starting to crust over.

Could he have gotten the chicken pox from the vaccine?

Yes, he could have. Some children who get vaccinated will still get the chicken pox, or will get it from the vaccine itself. Nicknamed "breakthrough chicken pox" by the medical community, these cases are usually minor. Most vaccinated children, however, will not experience any signs of the disease.

Is it contagious?

Yes. Chicken pox is very contagious and can easily spread from person to person by coughing, sneezing, or contact with the rash. The period during which people can catch the chicken pox from an infected person begins approximately two days prior to the rash breaking out and lasts until all of the blisters are crusted over.

Even if the chicken pox is a "breakthrough case," and the result of a vaccination, the rash is still contagious until all of the blisters are dried up and crusted over. Parents who have never had the chicken pox or who have never been vaccinated are most susceptible.

How common is the chicken pox?

It's not nearly as common as it used to be. The vaccination, which was approved for use in the United States in 1995, dramatically reduced the number of cases in our country. Some pediatricians have never even seen a live case of the chicken pox! Most American adults have already been exposed to the chicken pox or have had the vaccine and are therefore immune. But if an adult gets the chicken pox, the symptoms, including fever, malaise, and blisters, tend to be more severe. Adults also have a higher risk of complications, including pneumonia. Therefore, anyone who has not had the chicken pox or the vaccine should consider getting immunized.

It is worth mentioning that other once common childhood illnesses such as measles, mumps, and rubella have also experienced a dramatic decline due to routine vaccinations, and as a result, cases have become quite rare in the US.

Can you get it twice?

Technically yes, but it is very rare. For the vast majority of people, once you get it, you're immune.

It is important to realize that the virus that causes the chicken pox, known as varicella-zoster, remains in the body for life, usually in an inactive form. However, it can later get reactivated and produce a painful rash known as *shingles.* Shingles is more common in older people and can erupt in times of stress or illness, when the immune system is compromised. A person with shingles can give the chicken pox to another person who has never been exposed to the varicella-zoster virus.

Are there special concerns for pregnant women?

Pregnant women who have already had the chicken pox or received the vaccine do not need to be concerned.

Pregnant women who have not been exposed to the chicken pox should be careful. Studies have shown that both the mother and the fetus can experience serious complications, including birth defects for the baby, especially if the mom is exposed in the first five months of pregnancy.

Women who are unsure if they've been exposed to the chicken pox should consult a physician before getting pregnant. Any woman who thinks she has been exposed during her pregnancy and who is not immune, should also seek medical attention.

What is the treatment?

Chicken pox is usually treated at home with remedies that don't cure it but do lessen the symptoms. Medications such as acetaminophen or ibuprofen can be used to reduce the fever. Cold, damp compresses, oatmeal baths, and calamine lotion can reduce itchiness. If blisters are present in the mouth or throat, a bland-food or liquid diet may be recommended to relieve tenderness or discomfort. Antiviral medications such as acyclovir may also help lessen symptoms and are often recommended for patients with chronic diseases, adults, and other high-risk groups. Check with your doctor.

How can you lessen the chances of spreading the chicken pox?

The vaccination has done a great job reducing the number of chicken pox cases in our communities. Getting immunized is extremely effective in lessening the spread of the disease. Most doctors recommend that children get vaccinated between twelve and eighteen months. The US Centers for Disease Control and Prevention (CDC) recommends that every healthy adult without a known history of chicken pox also be vaccinated, so if you haven't had the vaccine, discuss it with your doctor.

Try to limit exposure to anyone who has an active case of the chicken pox or shingles and speak to your health care provider about additional ways to safeguard your household.

STOMACH FLU

You've tried everything: Cheerios, cut-up melon, even ice cream, but your one-year-old has no appetite. No matter what you serve, he throws it on the floor. He has a low-grade fever, but otherwise seems fine—until you change his diaper and notice that he has loose stools. He continues to have diarrhea throughout the day and, just when you're thinking this couldn't get any worse, he starts vomiting. You call the pediatrician who tells you the stomach flu is going around and there's nothing you can do for him except make sure to keep him hydrated. You shove a cherry popsicle in his mouth and hope for the best.

After you change diaper #6, the phone rings and you run for it, forgetting to wash your hands. *Whatever,* you think. *Who has time to wash their hands?* The next day, you feel nauseous and start to have stomach cramps. *No way, this can't be happening,* you think. But your thoughts are interrupted by having to race to the bathroom to vomit (for the first of what will turn out to be six times that day). You also have diarrhea for the next few days, until you and your son emerge from your ordeal five days later, weak but healthy—and three pounds lighter.

What caused this to happen?

The culprit: the stomach flu, which can be caused by a number of different viruses. It is very common in kids and is also highly contagious. Most moms and dads get it through close contact with their infected kids—for example, sharing food, beverages, and utensils, or handling soiled diapers.

What are the symptoms?

In young children, a loss of appetite may signal the start of the stomach flu. Remember, little kids who don't yet speak have a difficult time letting you know that their stomach hurts. So a sudden loss of appetite may be the only warning you will get that diarrhea and/or vomiting are on their way. (It's probably not the best time for you to finish the half-eaten grapes your child has left on the tray.)

In grown-ups, the most common symptoms of the stomach flu include: indigestion, nausea, loss of appetite, low-grade fever, stomach pain and cramps, diarrhea, and vomiting.

Are there any serious risks with the stomach flu?

Not really. Most people recover with no problems. But it is very important to stay hydrated. Young children and busy moms are both at risk of dehydration—children because they don't know they're supposed to drink, and you because you're busy and distracted. Repeated bouts of diarrhea and vomiting cause a significant loss of fluid from the body, which needs to be replaced.

Infants and young children can become easily dehydrated, so watch for these red flags:

- lethargy, or listless behavior
- little to no urine production (dry diapers)
- dry mouth
- decreased or no tears when crying
- sunken fontanelle (soft spot on an infant's head)

If your child experiences any of these warning signs, contact a doctor. It's important to note that the vast majority of kids with the stomach flu recover without becoming dehydrated.

The warning signs for dehydration in grown-ups include:

- increased thirst
- dry mouth, swollen tongue
- dizziness
- lethargy or weakness
- increased heart rate or palpitations (when your heart skips a beat)
- decreased production of urine or urine that is dark yellow in color

I have known several mothers who had to be hospitalized for dehydration because they didn't take the time to drink. So don't neglect yourself. Beverages with electrolytes, like Gatorade, are excellent options. Stay hydrated!

I know it may seem unthinkable to put something back down your throat while you have the stomach flu, but it is vital to do so. And at least you understand why you need to drink. Think of your poor child who can't understand why he is being forced to ingest watermelon-flavored Pedialyte at a time like this!

How can I lower my chances of getting the stomach flu from my child?

Wash your hands with soap and water. As simple as it sounds, it is the best way to avoid catching the stomach flu. Don't just rinse quickly, either. Really scrub your hands for at least ten to fifteen seconds, especially after changing a diaper. It may be hard to constantly wash your hands after changing a multitude of diapers. But just think of it this way: Would you rather spend the time washing your hands seven times or crouched over the toilet bowl vomiting seven times? That was an easy one!

Also, avoid sharing food with your child. Avoid sharing forks and spoons too. And no kissing! You may want to completely clean and disinfect with Clorox, or other related products, any surface (toilet bowl, changing table, highchair tray, car seat) which has been vomited on. Make sure to fully wrap and discard soiled diapers as well, keeping the surrounding area clean. This will help minimize the chances that you or another family member will catch the stomach flu.

LICE

When you went to pick up your three-year-old at preschool, there was a sign posted on the classroom door explaining that there was a case of lice in the school. When she saw you arrive, the director came out of her office with an information sheet from the doctor, which she handed out to everyone as they left with their children.

What are lice?

Lice are tiny, parasitic insects that live in human hair follicles and feed on minuscule amounts of blood from a person's scalp. It is a common problem, especially among school-age children. Girls seem to get head lice more often than boys, according to data from the Centers for Disease Control and Prevention. African-American children have the lowest risk when compared to other groups.

Are lice contagious?

Very! Anyone who comes in close contact with a child who has lice can catch it. Lice infestations are common in group settings, especially at schools, day care centers, playgrounds, and summer camps.

Family members are at risk as well, and not just siblings—Mom and Dad too! The risk of transmission is highest if there has been head-to-head contact (for example, sharing pillows, towels, hats, brushes, and combs, or lying on carpets, stuffed animals, or blankets). It should be noted that cats and dogs *cannot* catch or give head lice to human members of the family.

Are lice dangerous?

Head lice are not dangerous to a person's health and cannot transmit disease. But they can make a person pretty uncomfortable. Lice bites itch, so if a child is infected, you'll notice a lot of scratching. Sometimes, the bites can get red and swollen. It's important to look for signs of infection: red, tender skin and oozing from the bite sites.

How can you tell if you or your child has lice?

The itching and scratching will usually give it away, but some cases are fairly mild. Lice can often be seen if you examine the scalp. You may be able to see the eggs or nits at the base of the hair shaft, near the scalp, or you may spot the adult lice, which are no larger than sesame seeds and tend to congregate behind the ears and near the neck at the back of the head.

What is the treatment? Is it the same for kids and adults?

If you think you or your child has an infection, it needs to be addressed promptly. Lice can be treated with special nonprescription medicated shampoos or lotions. Speak with your doctor, because the type of medication used may vary, especially if the lice in your area have developed resistance to certain drugs. In these cases, your doctor may need to prescribe stronger medications.

Children and adults can be treated with the same type of medicated shampoo, cream, or lotion. But because most shampoos and lotions contain strong chemicals, some doctors do not recommend treating children under the age of two.

Removing lice by hand is usually suggested as the first-line treatment for children under two. Manual removal is recommended in wet hair, using a fine-toothed comb to physically remove the lice. Look along the entire hair shaft, because lice tend to lay eggs near the scalp and those need to be removed as well. The process should be repeated every few days for at least two weeks.

You should only treat yourself or other family members if you have been infested. It is *not* necessary to treat as a preventative measure. Just keep an eye out for the symptoms, and treat if need be.

How can you prevent lice from infecting others or coming back?

Here are a few tips for preventing lice from spreading or re-infecting family members:

- Wash all clothes, bed linens, and towels from the infected person separately, in hot water, and dry thoroughly in a heated dryer.
- Make sure to wash stuffed animals, throw pillows, etc., in hot water or send to the dry cleaner. If you cannot wash properly, you may want to discard.
- Throw out barrettes, headbands, brushes, or combs. If you want to keep them, make sure to soak in rubbing alcohol for at least an hour. Unless the item has sentimental value, it's better to chuck it.

- Vacuum all carpets, rugs, and furniture. (Don't forget to wash the car-seat cover!)
- Encourage family members to avoid sharing bike helmets, pillows, sleeping bags, combs, brushes, etc., with others.

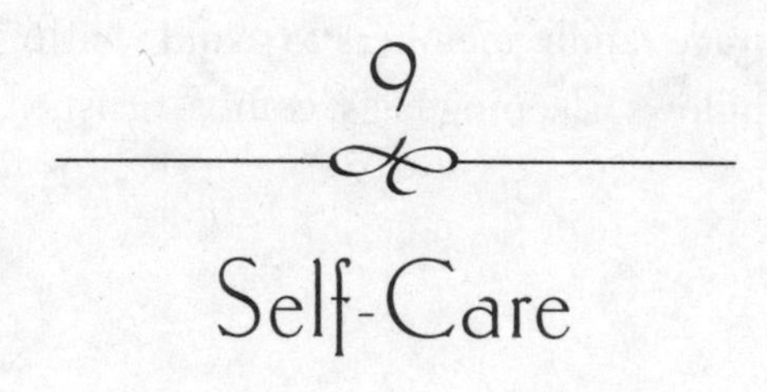

9
Self-Care

It's funny. We obsess about our health before and during pregnancy. Are we exercising enough? Are we eating a healthy diet? We see the doctor regularly and get dozens of tests—blood pressure, blood sugar, urinalysis, blood type, rubella, hepatitis and HIV screens, etc.—to make sure our bodies are disease-free and functioning well. Our friends, parents, husbands, in-laws, and mailmen all ask us how we are feeling on a daily basis. Everyone seems to care.

And then, we have the baby. We're sore, tired, worn-down, and, just when we need it the most . . . no one seems to care. And we have no time to take care of ourselves, either. We've gone from the top of the ladder of priorities to the lowest possible rung! We glance in the mirror and see dark circles under our eyes and flab on our bodies. We can't remember when we last went to the gym, saw the dentist, or had a haircut, and as the weeks turn into months, we forget to make an appointment with the gynecologist, too.

Who has time? Between the sleepless nights, grocery store runs, hard-to-please boss, hard-to-please newborn, carpooling, and pediatrician appointments, how can any of us remember to schedule our own doctor's appointments. . . .

Okay, so where does all of this leave us? In a not-so-good place, as far as our health is concerned. Studies have repeatedly demonstrated that women are the primary caretakers for their children, their aging parents, and their husbands—but often at their own expense.

Just because the baby is born doesn't mean we should neglect our own health. So many women wonder why they feel so exhausted and why they can't shed those extra pounds after pregnancy. But the problems go far beyond exhaustion and excess weight. I've spoken to women who have walked around for weeks with undiagnosed urinary tract infections, strep throat, viral pneumonia, and Lyme disease, ignoring the signs and symptoms because "they didn't have the time" to see a doctor.

For so many of us, our need to multitask, to take care of everyone else's needs, and run the household, in addition to handling all the other responsibilities we have, has precluded taking care of ourselves. So here I am, standing on a soapbox—telling you to make the time! Schedule your doctors' appointments; mark the dates on your calendar, and go! Even if you're not accustomed to putting yourself first, justify it by remembering how important your health and well-being are to the health and well-being of your entire family.

Screening

When asked what disease they fear the most, the overwhelming majority of women answer breast cancer, according to a survey commissioned by the Society for Women's Health Research, a nonprofit advocacy organization based in Washington, DC. Breast cancer tops the list despite the fact that heart disease is, by far, the number-one killer of women in the United States. More women will die from heart disease than from breast and all other gynecological cancers combined.

The risk of breast cancer should never be ignored, and proper preventative measures and screenings need to be in place for every woman. But there are other diseases out there that women need to be aware of—and heart disease isn't the only one.

Here are some facts that may surprise you:

- Heart disease kills roughly 500,000 American women annually and tends to strike women, on average, ten years later than men.
- Skin cancer is the most common cancer among men and women in this country.
- Lung cancer is the number-one cancer killer of women.
- Colon cancer is the third most common cancer among women, but many women with whom I spoke were under the impression that colorectal disease was a "man's disease."
- Osteoporosis, a disease distinguished by the loss of bone mass, affects women much more frequently than

men, necessitating proper dietary and nutritional choices for women from early on in their lives.

- Depression and anxiety disorders are two to three times more common in women than in men.
- Women are more likely to be obese than men, and because obesity is a major risk factor for diabetes, here's another disease to put on your radar screen.

What can I do to protect myself?

There's a lot you can do to safeguard your own health. Depending on your age, proper prevention, including doctors' visits and screening exams, tops the list of important things you can do for yourself. In addition, knowing your family's medical history is crucial. Sometimes, if certain diseases run in a particular family, doctors will recommend earlier and/or additional screening tests.

So when you visit the doctor, share your personal and family medical history, speak up, and ask questions. So many women are used to being the mouthpiece for everyone else in the family, often forgetting about themselves. Don't fall into this trap. Pay attention to your own health and make your appointments now. You're important too!

SCREENING TESTS FOR MOM

The following are a list of health care suggestions to guide you. Remember, not everyone in the medical community agrees on which tests are appropriate, so it is best to consult your own physician. Sometimes the screening exam guidelines will change depending on your personal history and your family's medical history. This is a general list for the average woman with normal risk factors.

If You Are a Younger Mom (Age 18–39)

- **Annual physical exam:** including blood pressure, cholesterol screening, height, weight, urine analysis, and clinical breast exam. If you have a history of gestational diabetes, blood glucose levels should be monitored by your physician. In addition, starting at the age of 35, you should also request thyroid screening, which involves a simple blood test.
- **Monthly breast self-exam:** to be performed a few days after your period ends. If you are breastfeeding and your period hasn't resumed, just pick a day—the same day each month—to do it. If you don't know how to do a breast self-exam, ask your doctor to walk you through it. Some offices have three-dimensional models that you can practice on and written materials that you can take home.
- **Pap smear and pelvic exam:** should be performed annually. New tests are available, including the HPV (human papillomavirus) test, which can identify the virus that causes cervical cancer. In addition, the HPV vaccine is currently recommended for girls and women ages 9–26. You may want to check in with your health care provider about guidelines for use of the HPV vaccine, which could change in the future. If you have new

or multiple sexual partners, you should also request STD (sexually transmitted disease) testing.

- **Skin exam:** annual skin exam by dermatologist to screen for skin cancer. If you have a family history of skin cancer, discuss with your doctor.
- **Dental exam:** annual oral-health exam and teeth cleaning by dentist. Some oral-health professionals recommend a cleaning and exam twice a year.
- **Make sure all of your immunizations are up-to-date:** Adults should check medical records to ensure that they were adequately immunized as children and should discuss additional vaccines against pneumococcal infection, influenza, and hepatitis B with their health care provider.

If You Are a Mom Age 40–49

- **Annual physical exam:** including blood pressure, cholesterol screening, height, weight, urine analysis, and clinical breast exam. Starting at the age of 45, blood glucose levels should be taken to screen for diabetes, and, if normal, they should be repeated every three years. Thyroid screening starts at the age of 35 and should be done every five years. In addition, if you have a history of heart disease in your family, discuss potential screening tests, including an exercise stress test or stress ECG.
- **Monthly breast self-exam:** to be performed a few days after your period ends. If your period is erratic, pick a day (for example the first day) to perform the exam and do it on the same day each month.

- **Mammogram:** The American Cancer Society recommends an annual mammogram for all women starting at the age of 40. If you have a family history of breast cancer, speak with your doctor. She may recommend starting mammograms earlier and/or using additional screening tests, including digital sonography.
- **Pap smear and pelvic exam:** should be performed annually. New tests are available, including the HPV (human papillomavirus) test, which can identify the virus that can cause cervical cancer. The HPV test has been approved for routine screening in women 30 years or older. If you have new or multiple sexual partners, you should also request STD (sexually transmitted disease) testing.
- **Skin exam:** annual skin exam by dermatologist to screen for skin cancer. If you have a family history of skin cancer, discuss with your doctor.
- **Dental exam:** annual oral-health exam and teeth cleaning by dentist. Some oral-health professionals recommend a cleaning and exam twice a year.
- **Make sure all of your immunizations are up-to-date.**

If You Are an Older Mom (50 Years and Up)

See all of the screenings for moms ages 40–49 and add these:

- **Annual fecal occult blood test:** to screen for colorectal disease.
- **Colonoscopy:** Begin screening at the age of 50 and repeat every ten years. Some doctors recommend

alternative screening tools, including flexible sigmoidoscopy or double-contrast barium enema, but studies have shown colonoscopy to be the most effective screening tool for colorectal cancer in women. If you have colorectal cancer in your family, speak with your doctor. You may require earlier screening and/or additional tests.

- **Eye exam:** every two to four years.
- **Hearing test:** every three years.
- **Bone health:** If you have osteoporosis in your family, speak with your doctor about assessing your bone health and what you can do to prevent bone disease. Routine screening for osteoporosis in average-risk women is not officially recommended in this age group, but if you're concerned, speak with your doctor.
- **Lung health:** researchers continue to look for more effective ways to prevent and screen for lung cancer. Currently, chest X-rays, CT scans, and sputum cytology (looking for cancer cells in phlegm under a microscope), are among the available screening tools. Studies reveal that these tools have varying degrees of accuracy, and may result in false positives that then require costly and invasive follow-up testing, so doctors are divided about which of them, if any, should be used. Discuss with your health care provider, especially if you have a history of smoking or family history of lung cancer.

AFTERWORD

Becoming a new mother is like no other experience you will ever have. Your life has suddenly become full of wonderful changes, but you'll definitely be facing some brand-new challenges, and taking on a lot of new responsibilities, too.

Women typically become the primary caretakers of their families. It is we who make the doctor appointments for our children, our partners, and sometimes even our parents—while often forgetting to make them for ourselves. We wipe runny noses, dole out medications and vitamins, sleep standing up, and call colleagues from the car between day care pickups, music classes, and supermarket runs. We make Wonder Woman look lazy. But almost no one, except maybe our own mothers, ever notices how brilliantly we are managing everything and everyone—everyone except ourselves, that is.

All these challenges take a huge toll on us, so that at the

end of the day we're exhausted, but because we are accustomed to putting ourselves at the bottom of our priority list, we tend to ignore our own physical, psychological, sexual, and emotional needs. If we're lucky, we may be able to fit in a little bedtime reading before we collapse onto our pillows, but even that is more likely to be an article on homemade baby food or common childhood rashes rather than the latest book everyone is talking about.

Unfortunately, ignoring ourselves until our minds and our bodies give off not-so-subtle hints that they are in trouble is not going to do anyone any good, because our families need us to be strong and healthy. Whatever the problem, whether it's something as relatively minor as difficulty losing weight or as major as postpartum depression or diabetes, we should make sure that our needs are addressed—and sooner, rather than later, before small problems become big ones.

Being a good mother involves taking care of ourselves and recognizing when we need some rest, some extra help and support, some private time, or some medical attention. The journey of motherhood is filled with the greatest thrills and the deepest, most selfless love in the world, but selflessness must not be confused with self-denial or self-destruction. We must discover a balance that allows us to fulfill our obligations to those we love while also accommodating our own needs as women, partners, and mothers. Our families will be better for it.

BIBLIOGRAPHY

Albani, S., and D. A. Carson. A multistep molecular mimicry hypothesis for the pathogenesis of rheumatoid arthritis. *Immunol Today*. 1996;17:466–70.

Albers, L. L., Sedler, K. D., and E. J. Bedrick. Factors related to genital tract trauma in normal spontaneous vaginal births. *Birth*. 2006 Jun;33(2):94–100.

Alder, E. M., Cook, A., Davidson, D., West, C., and J. Bancroft. Hormones, mood and sexuality in lactating women. *Br J Psychiatry*. 1986 Jan;148:74–9.

American Academy of Pediatrics. Committee on Infectious Diseases. Varicella vaccine update. *Pediatrics*. 2000 Jan;105(1 Pt 1):136–41. Review.

Avery, M. D., Duckett, L., and C. R. Frantzich. The experience of sexuality during breastfeeding among primiparous women. *J Midwifery Womens Health*. 2000;45:227–36.

Ayoob, K. T., and R. L. Duyff. Position of the American Dietetic Association: food and nutrition misinformation. *J Am Diet Assoc*. 2002 Feb;102(2):260–6.

Beers, M. H., and R. S. Porter (eds). *The Merck Manual*, 18th Ed. Merck & Co., Inc., 2006.

Behnauskiene, J. Glucose tolerance of 2- to 5-yr-old offspring of diabetic mothers. *Pediatr Diabetes.* 2004 Sep;5(3):143–6.

Bellantuono, C., et al. Serotonin reuptake inhibitors in pregnancy and the risk of major malformations: a systematic review. *Hum Psychopharmacol.* 2007 Apr;22(3):121–8.

Belsky, J., and K. H. Hsieh. Patterns of marital change during the early childhood years: parent personality, coparenting and division of labor correlates. *Journal of Family Psychology.* 1998 Dec;12(4):511–28.

Berle, J. O., Steen, V. M., Aamo, T. O., et al. Breastfeeding during maternal antidepressant treatment with serotonin reuptake inhibitors: infant exposure, clinical symptoms, and cytochrome p450 genotypes. *J Clin Psychiatry.* 2004 Sep;65(9):1228–34.

Bradley, C. S., Kennedy, C. M., et al. Pelvic floor symptoms and lifestyle factors in older women. *J Womens Health.* 2005 Mar;14(2):128–36.

Brent, N., et al. Sore nipples in breastfeeding women: a clinical trial of wound dressings vs. conventional care. *Arch Pediatric Adolesc Med.* 1998 Nov;152:1077–82.

Britton, J. R. Maternal anxiety: course and antecedents during the early postpartum period. *Depress Anxiety.* Mar 30, 2007.

Broliden, K., Tolfvenstam, T., and O. Norbeck. Clinical aspects of parvovirus B19 infection. *J Intern Med.* 2006 Oct;260(4):285–304.

Buckwalter, J. G., et al. Pregnancy and post partum: changes in cognition and mood. *Prog Brain Res.* 2001;133:303–19.

Burt, V. K., and K. Stein. Epidemiology of depression throughout the female life cycle. *J Clin Psychiatry.* 2002;63(Suppl 7):9–15.

Byrd, J. E., Hyde, J. S., DeLamater, J. D., and E. A. Plant. Sexuality during pregnancy and the year postpartum. *J Fam Pract.* 1998;47:305–08.

Cable, B., Stewart, M., and J. Davis. Nipple wound care: a new approach to an old problem. *J Hum Lact.* 1997 Dec;13(4):313–18.

Chaudron, L. H., and R. W. Pies. The relationship between postpartum psychosis and bipolar disorder: a review. *J Clin Psychiatry.* 2003 Nov;64(11):1284–92.

Chunge, R.N., Scott, F. E., Underwood J. E., and K. J. Zavarella. A pilot study to investigate transmission of head lice. *Can J Public Health.* 1991;82: 207–08.

Cowan, P. A., and C. P. Cowan. Changes in marriage during the transition to parenthood: must we blame the baby? *The Transition to Parenthood: Current Theory and Research,* ed. G. Y. Michaels and W. A. Goldberg. New York: Cambridge University Press, 1988.

Cox, J. Postnatal depression in fathers. *Lancet.* 2005 Sep 17–23;366(9490):982.

Cram, Sally, DDS, American Dental Association. Interview June 28, 2006.

Cunningham, F. G., Leveno, K., et al. *Williams Obstetrics, 22nd edition.* New York: McGraw-Hill, 2005.

Dewey, K. Effects of maternal caloric restriction and exercise during lactation. *Journal of Nutrition.* 1998 Feb;128 (2): 386S–389S.

Diseases most feared by women, survey—International Communications Research of Media, Pa., for the Society for Women's Health Research, 2005 June 22–29.

Donnelly, V., Fynes, M., Campbell, D., Johnson, H., O'Connell, P. R., and C. O'Herlihy. Obstetric events leading to anal sphincter damage. *Obstet Gynecol.* 1998;92:955–61.

Duffy, L. Breastfeeding after strenuous aerobic exercise: a case report. *J Hum Lact.* 1997 Jun;13(2):145–6.

Dzaja, A., Arber, S., Hislop, J., et al. Women's sleep in health and disease. *J Psychiatr Res.* 2005 Jan;39(1):55–76.

Epperson, C. N. Postpartum major depression: detection and treatment. *American Family Physician.* 1999 April 15; Vol. 59/No. 8.

Forster, C., Abraham, S., Taylor, A., D. Llewellyn-Jones. Psychological and sexual changes after the cessation of breast-feeding. *Obstet Gynecol.* 1994;84:872–876.

Gabbe, S., Hill, L., Schmidt, L., et al. Management of diabetes by obstetricians and gynecologists. *Obstet Gynecol.* 1998; 91:643.

Garner, P. Type 1 diabetes and pregnancy. *Lancet.* 346:157, 1995b.

Gay, C. L., Lee, K. A., and S. Y. Lee. Sleep patterns and fatigue in new mothers and fathers. *Biol Res Nurs.* 2004 Apr;5(4): 311–18.

Geerts, S. O., Legrand, V., et al. Further evidence of the association between periodontal conditions and coronary artery disease. *J Periodontol.* 2004 Sep;75(9):1274–80.

Giugliani, E. R. Common problems during lactation and their management. *J Pediatr (Rio J).* 2004 Nov;80(5 Suppl):S147–54.

Grimes, P. Incidence and psychosocial implications of melasma. Presented at: American Academy of Dermatology; July 25–29, 2003; Chicago, Ill.

Hackel, L. S., and D. N. Ruble. Changes in the marital relationship after the first baby is born: predicting the impact of expectancy disconfirmation. *J Pers Soc Psychol.* 1992 Jun;62(6):944–57.

Hartmann, K., Viswanathan, M., et al. Outcomes of routine episiotomy: a systematic review. *JAMA.* 2005; 293: 2141–48.

Hudelist, G., Gelle'n, J., and C. Singer. Factors predicting severe perineal trauma during childbirth: role of forceps delivery routinely combined with mediolateral episiotomy. *Am J Obstet Gynecol.* 2005 Mar;192(3):875–81.

Jeffcoat, M. K., Geurs, N. C., Reddy, M. S., et al. Periodontal infection and preterm birth: results of a prospective study. *J Am Dent Assoc.* 2001 Jul;132(7):875–80.

Kennedy, K., and C. Visness. Contraceptive efficacy of lactational amenorrhoea. *Lancet.* 1992; 339: 227–29.

Kinlay, J. R., O'Connell, D. L., and S. Kinlay. Risk factors for mastitis in breastfeeding women: results of a prospective cohort study. *Aust N Z J Pub Health.* 2001 Apr;25(2):115–20.

Kocić B., Petrović B., and S. Janković. Diet and breast cancer. *J BUON.* 2003 Jul–Sep;8(3):221–28.

Lee, K. Y., et al. Diverse developmental toxicity of di-n-butyl phthalate in both sexes of rat offspring after maternal exposure during the period from late gestation through lactation. *Toxicology.* 2004 Oct 15;203(1–3):221–38.

Lukacz, E. S., Lawrence, J. M., Contreras, R., et al. Parity, mode of delivery, and pelvic floor disorders. *Obstet Gynecol.* 2006 Jun;107(6):1253–60.

Marcus, S., Barry, K., et al. Depressive symptoms among pregnant women screened in obstetrics settings. *J Women's Health.* 2003 May;12(4):373–80.

Melo, S. B., and M. I. Fernandes. Prevalence and demographic characteristics of celiac disease among blood donors in Ribeirao Preto, State of São Paulo, Brazil. *Dig Dis Sci.* 2006 May;51(5):1020–25. Epub 2006 Jun 7.

Mohammadzadeh, A., Farhat, A., and H. Esmaeily. The effect of breast milk and lanolin on sore nipples. *Saudi Med J.* 2005 Aug;26(8):1231–34.

Mohrbacher, N., and J. Stock. *The Breastfeeding Answer Book* (Third Revised Edition). La Leche League International, Schaumburg, Illinois, 2003.

Molitch, M. E. Pituitary disease in pregnancy. *Semin Perinatol.* 1998 Dec;22(6):457–70.

National Vital Statistics Report. 2004 Oct. 12;Vol. 53, No. 5.

Newport, D. J., Hostetter, A., Arnold, A., and Z. N. Stowe. The treatment of postpartum depression: minimizing infant exposures. *J Clin Psychiatry.* 2002;63(Suppl 7):33–44.

Okun, M. L., and M. E. Coussons-Read. Sleep disruption during pregnancy: How does it influence serum cytokines? *J Reprod Immunol.* 2006 Oct 27;73(2):158–65.

Oliveri, B., Parisi, M. S., Zeni, S., and C. Mautalen. Mineral and bone mass changes during pregnancy and lactation. *Nutrition.* 2004;20(2):235–40.

Paulson, S. E. Relations of parenting style and parental involvement with ninth-grade students' achievement. *Journal of Early Adolescence.* 1994;14(2):250–67.

Plourd, D. M., and K. Austin. Correlation of a reported history of chickenpox with seropositive immunity in pregnant women. *J Reprod Med.* 2005 Oct;50(10):779–83.

Pollack, J., Nordenstram, J., Brismar, S., et al. Anal incontinence after vaginal delivery: a five-year prospective cohort study. *Obstet Gynecol.* 2004;104:1397.

Pollack, R. J., Kiszewski, A. E., and A. Spielman. Overdiagnosis and consequent mismanagement of head louse infestations in North America. *Pediatr Infect Dis J.* 2000;19:689–93.

Reamy, K. J., and S. E. White. Sexuality in the puerperium: a review. *Arch Sex Behav.* 1987;16:165–86.

Rowland, M., Foxcroft, L., et al. Breastfeeding and sexuality immediately post partum. *Can Fam Physician.* 2005 Oct 10; 51(10):1367.

Saar, P., Hermann, W., and U. Muller-Ladner. Connective tissue diseases and pregnancy. *Rheumatology* (Oxford). 2006 Oct;45 (Suppl 3):iii30–iii32.

Samuelsson, E., Ladfors, L., Wennerholm, U. B., Gareberg, B., Nyberg, K., and H. Hagberg. Anal sphincter tears: prospective study of obstetric risk factors. *Br J Obstet Gynaecol.* 2000;107:926–31.

Scheithauer, B. W., Sano, T., Kovacs, K. T., et al. The pituitary gland in pregnancy: A clinicopathologic and immunohistochemical study of 69 cases. *Mayo Clin Proc.* 1990 Apr;65(4):461–74.

Schoenfeld, P., et al. Colonoscopic screening of average-risk women for colorectal neoplasia. *N Engl J Med.* 2005; 352: 2061–68.

Seldin, M. F., Amos, C. I., Ward, R., and P. K. Gregerson. The genetics revolution and the assault on rheumatoid arthritis. *Arthritis Rheum.* 1999;42:1071–79.

Sit, D., Rothschild, A. J., and K. L. Wisner. A review of postpartum psychosis. *J Womens Health.* 2006 May;15(4):352–68.

Steiner, M. Perinatal mood disorders: position paper. *Psychopharmacol Bull.* 1998;34(3):301–6.

Steiner, M. Postpartum psychiatric disorders. *Can J Psychiatry.* 1990;35:89–95.

Thurtle, V. Post-natal depression: the relevance of sociological approaches. *J Adv Nurs.* 1995;22(3):416–24.

US Department of Agriculture Dietary Guidelines. Available from: http://www.health.gov/DietaryGuidelines.

Way, C. M. Safety of newer antidepressants in pregnancy. *Pharmacotherapy*. 2007 Apr;27(4):546–52.

Webber, V., and M. Zahorick. Postpartum body image and weight loss. *New Beginnings*. 2000 Sept–Oct;17(6):45,156–59.

Weissman, M., et al. Remissions in maternal depression and child psychopathology. *JAMA*. 2006;295:1389–98.

Whitton, A., Warner, R., and L. Appleby. The pathway to care in post-natal depression: women's attitudes to post-natal depression and its treatment. *Br J Gen Pract*. 1996 Jul;46(408):427–28.

Xu, J., Eilat-Adar, S., Loria, C., et al. Dietary fat intake and risk of coronary heart disease: the strong heart study. *Am J Clin Nutr*. 2006 Oct;84(4):894–902.

Yonkers, K. A., and S. J. Chantilis. Recognition of depression in obstetric/gynecology practices. *Am J Obstet Gynecol*. 1995; 173(2):632–38.

Young, G. L., and D. Jewell. Creams for preventing stretch marks in pregnancy (Cochrane Review). In: The Cochrane Library, Issue 3, 2003. Oxford: Update Software.

INDEX

ABOUT THE AUTHOR

JENNIFER WIDER, MD, is a doctor, author, and radio personality who specializes in women's health issues. She is the medical advisor to the Society for Women's Health Research in Washington, D.C. Dr. Wider is a regular contributor to *Cosmopolitan* magazine and hosts a weekly segment on Cosmo Radio for Sirius Satellite. She has appeared as a health expert on *The Today Show, CBS News, Good Day NY, Fox News*, and a variety of cable channels. She lives with her physician husband, and their daughter and son, in Fairfield County, Connecticut.